Health Framework for California Public Schools

Kindergarten Through Grade Twelve

Developed by the
Curriculum Development and Supplemental
Materials Commission

Adopted by the
California State Board of Education

Published by the
California Department of Education

Publishing Information

When the *Health Framework for California Public Schools: Kindergarten Through Grade Twelve* was adopted by the California State Board of Education on March 6, 2002, the members of the State Board were the following: Reed Hastings, President; Joe Nuñez, Vice-President; Robert Abernethy; Donald G. Fisher; Susan Hammer; Nancy Ichinaga; Carlton Jenkins; Marion Joseph; Vicki Reynolds; Suzanne Tacheny; and Erika Goncalves.

The framework was developed by the Curriculum Development and Supplemental Materials Commission. (See pages vi–xi for the names of the members of the commission and the names of the principal writers and others who made significant contributions to the framework.)

This publication was edited by Dixie Abbott, working in cooperation with Greg Geeting, Assistant Executive Director, State Board of Education, and Thomas Adams, Director, Thomas Akin, Consultant, and Christopher Dowell, Consultant, Curriculum Frameworks and Instructional Resources Division, California Department of Education. It was designed and prepared for printing by the staff of CDE Press, with the cover and interior design created and prepared by Cheryl McDonald. Typesetting was done by Jeannette Huff. The framework was published by the Department of Education, 1430 N Street, Sacramento, California (mailing address: P.O. Box 944272, Sacramento, CA 94244-2720). It was distributed under the provisions of the Library Distribution Act and *Government Code* Section 11096.

ISBN 0-8011-1574-4

Ordering Information

Copies of this publication are available for $17.50 each, plus shipping and handling charges. California residents are charged sales tax. Orders may be sent to the California Department of Education, CDE Press, Sales Office, P.O. Box 271, Sacramento, CA 95812-0271; FAX (916) 323-0823. Prices on all publications are subject to change.

An illustrated *Educational Resources Catalog* describing publications, videos, and other instructional media available from the Department can be obtained without charge by writing to the address given above or by calling the Sales Office at (916) 445-1260 or (800) 995-4099.

Contents

Foreword

The California State Board of Education and the California Department of Education are pleased to present the 2003 edition of the *Health Framework for California Public Schools*, adopted by the State Board of Education on March 6, 2002. This edition contains the content of the 1994 framework and provides updated information on curriculum development, health literacy, positive asset development among youths, research-based programs, school safety, and special student populations.

In the years since the approval of the 1994 framework, educators have come to understand the importance of positive approaches to health education. Curriculum that is based on the updated framework will help students build strong relationships with their families and communities while strengthening their resiliency and personal decision-making skills for healthy living. Health education within the context of a coordinated school health program contributes to results such as decreased tobacco use and improved choices about nutrition and physical activity.

The framework includes an important change for teachers as it gives greater guidance on what should be taught at each grade level. At the end of Chapter 3, "Health Education," the Grade-Level Emphases Chart suggests specific topics to emphasize in each grade. Although the topics appeared in the 1994 edition, they have been placed in specific grades for the first time in this new edition.

While the 2003 framework reflects many positive developments in health education, it also addresses the concerns resulting from tragic events. Noteworthy are the updated discussions of school safety, mental health, and violence prevention. We cannot stress enough the need to make schools safe, free from intolerance, and a place for learning.

The framework has been strengthened by a discussion about research-based programs and the use of survey data. Rigorous criteria for evaluating programs, derived from the Centers for Disease Control and Prevention and the California Department of Education publication series *Getting Results,* are presented to give health educators the tools they need to select the most effective programs for educating students.

Good health, by definition, requires lifelong learning. A better life for our youths begins with teaching them from an early age how to be physically and mentally healthy.

JACK O'CONNELL
State Superintendent of Public Instruction

REED HASTINGS
President, State Board of Education

Acknowledgments

The *Health Framework for California Public Schools, Kindergarten Through Grade Twelve,* was adopted by the California State Board of Education on March 6, 2002. On October 7, 1999, the State Board of Education directed the California Department of Education and the Curriculum Development and Supplemental Materials Commission (Curriculum Commission) to retain the content of the 1994 framework while updating it with the development of sixteen health topics.* The names of the persons who contributed to the development of the *Health Framework,* starting with those who contributed to the 2003 edition, are as follows:

Health Framework (2003 edition)

The following persons served on the Curriculum Commission when the 2003 *Health Framework* was recommended to the State Board of Education on January 18, 2002:

Susan Stickel, Chair
Norma Baker
Catherine Banker
William Brakemeyer
Mary Coronado Calvario
Edith Crawford
Milissa Glen-Lambert
Lora L. Griffin
Sandra Mann
Veronica Norris
Leslie Schwarze
Dale Webster
Karen S. Yamamoto

Note: The titles and affiliations of persons named in this section were current at the time the document was developed.

* The following chapters contain the newly developed health topics: Chapter 1 (definitions of terms; schools and health; positive youth development, asset development, and resiliency; use of evaluation and survey data in school health programs; California's Healthy Start Initiative); Chapter 2 (importance of research-based programs; life skills and positive behaviors; health education planning and development; needs of special populations); Chapter 3 (scope and sequence of health instruction); and Chapter 4 (local advisory or coordinating councils; health services in schools; mental health issues in schools; the California public mental health system and schools; safe schools and violence prevention; suicide prevention).

Guidance for the development of the 2003 framework was provided by the Chair, Health Subject Matter Committee of the Curriculum Commission:

Veronica N. Norris, Tustin, California

Other members of the Health Subject Matter Committee were:

Roy Anthony, Valhalla High School, Grossmont Union High School District

Milissa Glen-Lambert, Monlux Elementary School, Los Angeles Unified School District

Lora L. Griffin, Retired Educator, Sacramento City Unified School District

Richard Schwartz, Torrance High School, Torrance Unified School District

Susan Stickel, Elk Grove Unified School District

Karen Yamamoto, Westmore Oaks Elementary School, Washington Unified School District

Coordination of the development of the 2003 framework was provided by:

Sherry Skelly Griffith, Assistant Superintendent, Curriculum Frameworks and Instructional Resources Division, California Department of Education; and Executive Secretary, Curriculum Commission

Thomas Adams, Administrator, Curriculum Frameworks and Instructional Resources Division, California Department of Education

The principal writer was **Hank Resnik.**

Coordination of content was provided by:

Jeri Day, Health Education Specialist, School Health Connections, California Department of Education

Caroline Roberts, Administrator, School Health Connections, California Department of Education

Chapter 3, "Health Education," contains the "Grade-Level Emphases Chart," developed in part by a focus group of educators in July 2001. Members of that focus group were:

Glenda Bensussen, Los Angeles Unified School District

Phyllis Camp, San Francisco Unified School District

Meri Fedak, Long Beach Unified School District

Tracy Harrington, Long Beach Unified School District

Jane Huston, Mount Shasta Unified School District

Robert LaChausse, California State University, San Bernardino

Tracy Parker, Galt Unified School District

Ann Rector, Long Beach Unified School District

Enrique Robles, Los Angeles Unified School District

Deborah Wood, Healthy Kids Resource Center

Contributions to the completion of the framework were made by the following staff members in the Curriculum Frameworks and Instructional Resources Division, California Department of Education:

Thomas Akin, Consultant

Christopher Dowell, Consultant

Teri Ollis, Staff Services Analyst

Tonya Odums, Support Staff

Lino Vicente, Support Staff

Beverly Wilson, Support Staff

Additional staff members from the California Department of Education who contributed to the completion of the framework were:

Jackie Allen, Counseling and Student Support Services

Donna Bezdecheck, School Health Connections

John Boivin, Educational Options

Linda Davis-Alldritt, School Health Connections

Rona Gordon, Child, Youth, and Family Services

Mary Lu Graham, Healthy Start and After-School Partnerships

Joanna Knieriem, School Health Connections

Jan Lewis, Nutrition Services

Vivian Linfor, Safe Schools and Violence Prevention

Karen Lowrey, Counseling and Student Support Services

John Malloy, Healthy Start and After School Partnerships

Doug McDougall, Healthy Start and After School Partnerships

Paul Meyers, Counseling and Student Support Service

Patricia Michael, Special Education

Roberta Peck, Healthy Start and After School Partnerships

Rachel Perry, Evaluation

Ronda Simpson-Brown, Youth Education Partnerships

Bill White, Safe Schools and Violence Prevention

Bonnie Williamson, Safe Schools and Violence Prevention

Milt P. Wilson, Retired Annuitant

Dianne Wilson-Graham, School Health Connections

Other contributors included:

Gregory Austin, Director, Health and Human Development Program, WestEd

Dave Neilsen, California Department of Mental Health

Jackie Russum, Healthy Kids Resource Center

Deborah Wood, Healthy Kids Resource Center

Health Framework (1994 edition)

Guidance for the development of the 1994 framework was provided by the Chair, Health Subject Matter Committee, Curriculum Commission:

Eugene Flores, Arroyo Grande High School, Lucia Mar Unified School District

The 1994 Health Curriculum Framework and Criteria Committee, composed of nine California health educators and health professionals, was chaired by:

Justin Cunningham, Healthy Kids Regional Center, Region IX, San Diego Office of Education

The other committee members were:

Claudia Baker, Los Angeles Unified School District

Diane Chagnon, Somerset Senior Elementary School, Sylvan Union Elementary School District

Linda Davis-Alldritt, Elk Grove Unified School District

Ellen Jones, Alameda County Office of Education

Shirley Knight-Lopez, Pajaro Valley Unified School District

Nathan Matza, Westminster High School, Huntington Beach Union High School District

Cornelia Owens, Los Angeles Unified School District

Marilyn Wells, Alhambra City Elementary and High School District

Coordination for the development, field review, and preparation of the 1994 framework was provided by:

Glen Thomas, Curriculum Frameworks and Instructional Resources Office, California Department of Education

The principal writer of the field-review version of the framework was **William Boly.**

Chapter 3 of the 1994 framework was based on preliminary work done by a committee of educators during 1989–90. Members of the model curriculum guide committee were:

Peter Cortese, California State University, Long Beach

Justin Cunningham, San Diego County Office of Education

Gus Dalis, Los Angeles County Office of Education

Margaret Leeds, Beverly Hills High School, Beverly Hills Unified School District

Ric Loya, California Association of School Health Educators

Pamela Luna, Riverside County Office of Education

Priscilla Naworski, Comprehensive Health Education Resource Center, Alameda County Office of Education

Staff support from the California Department of Education to the model curriculum guide committee was provided by:

Amanda Dew Manning, Healthy Kids, Healthy California Office

Jennifer Rousseve, Healthy Kids, Healthy California Office

Jacqui Smith, Healthy Kids, Healthy California Office

Detailed information for Chapter 3 was provided by:

Ruth Bowman, Washington Unified School District

Justin Cunningham, San Diego County Office of Education

Joan Davies, Alameda County Office of Education

Pamela Luna, Riverside County Office of Education

Priscilla Naworski, Comprehensive Health Education Resource Center, Alameda County Office of Education

Jean Varden, Ventura County Office of Education

The final stages of the development of the 1994 framework were directed by:

Justin Cunningham, San Diego County Office of Education

Ellen Jones, Alameda County Office of Education

Critical support was provided by:

Nancy Sullivan, Curriculum Frameworks and Instructional Resources Office, California Department of Education

The State Board of Education's liaisons to the Curriculum Commission, **Kathryn Dronenburg** and **Sark "Bill" Malkasian,** provided invaluable direction and support in the final stages of development of the framework.

The principal writer of the final version of the 1994 framework was **Hank Resnik.**

Staff support from the California Department of Education was provided by:

Ples Griffin, Health Promotion Office

Jennifer Rousseve, Healthy Kids, Healthy California Office

Robert Ryan, Healthy Kids, Healthy California Office

Nancy Sullivan, Curriculum Frameworks and Instructional Resources Office

In addition, many other persons in the California Department of Education provided assistance during the development process of the 1994 framework, most notably:

Janice DeBenedetti, Home Economics Education Unit

Mary Lu Graham, Migrant Education Program

Emily Nahat, Interagency Youth and Children Services

Dennis Parker, Categorical Programs Division

Roberta Peck, Nutrition and Food Service Education Section

Jacqui Smith, Healthy Kids, Healthy California Office

Janine Swanson, Special Education Division

Kathy Yeates, Healthy Kids, Healthy California Office

Members of the Health Subject Matter Committee of the Curriculum Commission responsible for overseeing the development of the 1994 framework, including the field review, were:

Del Alberti, Washington Unified School District

Gloria Blanchette, Sacramento Unified School District

Dan Chernow, Pacific Theaters Corporation, Los Angeles

Bruce Fisher, Fortuna Elementary School, Fortuna Union Elementary School District

Eugene Flores (Chair, 1992), Arroyo Grande High School, Lucia Mar Unified School District

Harriet Harris, Del Mar Elementary School, Fresno Unified School District

Charles Kloes, Beverly Hills High School, Beverly Hills Unified School District

Charles Koepke, Upland Junior High School, Upland Unified School District

Tom Vasta (Chair, 1991), Elk Grove Unified School District

Vivian Lee Ward, Sequoia High School, Sequoia Union High School District

We need to make a national commitment to health education that is far greater than the routine and merely ceremonial attention we usually give it. . . . We need to teach youngsters that they must take charge of their health—all of their lives. . . . And we must do more than teach; we must set an example in the way we live.

—C. Everett Koop, M.D.
Koop: The Memories of America's Family Doctor

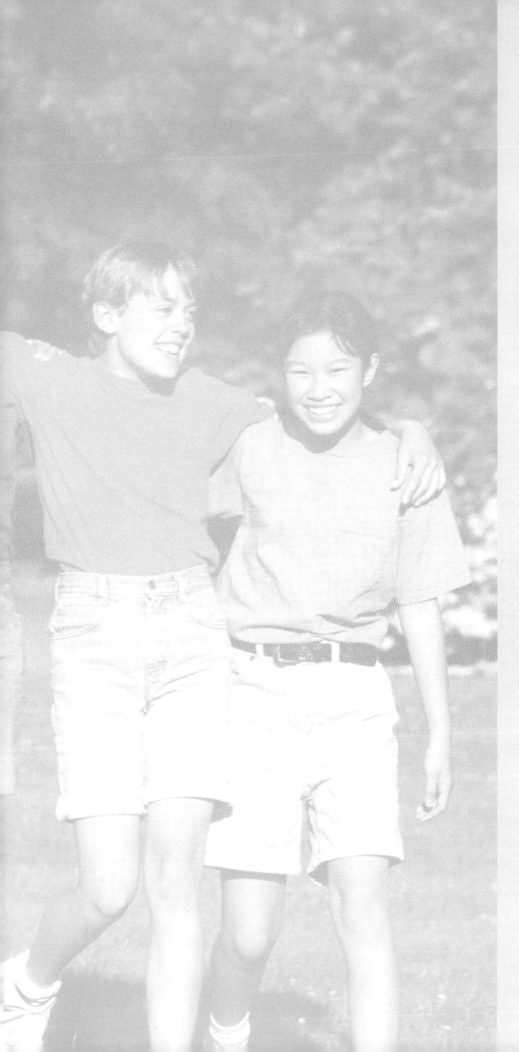

CHAPTER 1

The Vision:
Health Literacy,
Healthy Schools,
Healthy People

Emphasis must be
placed on developing
lifelong, positive health-
related attitudes and
behaviors.

Health literacy is "the
capacity of an individual
to obtain, interpret, and
understand basic health
information and services
and the competence to
use such information and
services in ways which
are health-enhancing."

—*Journal of Health
Education*

In recent decades Americans have successfully coped with serious health problems. Many diseases and illnesses, such as polio and diphtheria, that once threatened vast numbers of people can now be prevented or treated effectively. As a result, a growing percentage of the population is staying healthier and living longer. However, far too many children and youths die because of injuries that are unintentional or result from violent behavior, and others compromise their health through unhealthy behaviors, such as using alcohol, tobacco, or other drugs. In addition, diseases brought on by unhealthy behaviors often cause the premature deaths of adults. Responding to these health problems requires a commitment to health education. Individuals must understand the role they must play in protecting, maintaining, and promoting their health and the health of others through healthy behaviors and choices.

Two factors central to this new approach to health education are as follows:

- Emphasis must be placed on developing lifelong, positive health-related attitudes and behaviors. Such attitudes and behaviors begin to be developed in the home. But the school, working in close partnership with families and communities, is also an appropriate arena for development and reinforcement.[1]

- Health education in the schools must be supported by a comprehensive schoolwide system to promote children's health and must be developed and sustained by the collaborative efforts of school personnel, parents, school board members, community leaders, and health and social services agencies and providers.

When these elements are in place, children and youths can be helped to develop a lifelong commitment to their own health and well-being.

Throughout this framework the knowledge, skills, and behaviors needed for healthy living are referred to as health literacy. According to the Association for the Advancement of Health Education, health literacy is "the capacity of an individual to obtain, interpret, and understand basic health information and services and the competence to use such information and services in ways which are health-enhancing."[2] A health-literate person understands scientifically based principles of health promotion and disease prevention, incorporates that knowledge into personal health-related attitudes and behaviors, and makes good health a personal priority.

This framework is based on the premise that health literacy is as important in today's complex, challenging world as linguistic, mathematical, and scientific literacy. The major goal of this framework is to describe health education and schoolwide health promotion strategies that will help children and youths

---

[1] In this document the term *community* includes religious institutions, community leaders, businesses, health-care providers, and other agencies and organizations involved in children's development.

[2] "Report of the 1990 Joint Committee on Health Education Terminology," *Journal of Health Education*, Vol. 22, No. 2 (1991), 104.

become health-literate individuals with a lifelong commitment to healthy living.

Because every aspect of health is tangibly connected to life and students' experiences, effective health education provides abundant opportunities for engaging students in purposeful learning. Health-literate students will make a commitment to their own health and the health of others, enhancing school efforts to involve students in collaborative, meaningful learning experiences.

The following commonly used terms have been defined to facilitate the use of this framework. They were adapted from a report of the Association for the Advancement of Health Education and have been updated from the 1994 edition of the *Health Framework*.

Health. A state of complete physical, mental, and social well-being, not merely the absence of disease and infirmity.

Health literacy. The capacity of an individual to obtain, interpret, and understand basic health information and services and the competence to use such information and services in ways that are health-enhancing.

Coordinated school health system (updated term for *comprehensive school health system* as recommended in the books *Health Is Academic* and *Schools and Health*).[3] An organized set of policies, procedures, and activities developed and implemented through a collaborative effort that includes parents, the school, and the community. The system is designed to protect and promote the health and well being of students and staff. A coordinated school health system includes health education, physical education, health services, nutrition services, psychological and counseling services, a safe and healthy school environment, health promotion for staff, and parent and community involvement.

Health education. One component of a coordinated school health system. It includes the development, delivery, and evaluation of a planned, sequential curriculum for students in kindergarten through grade twelve and for parents and school staff and is designed to influence positively people's knowledge, attitudes, skills, and behaviors related to health. Health education addresses the four unifying ideas of health literacy and the following nine content areas: personal health; consumer and community health; injury prevention and safety; alcohol, tobacco, and other drugs; nutrition; environmental health; family living; individual growth and development; and communicable and chronic diseases.

Health education focused on developing health literacy through a student centered curriculum will enhance school-reform efforts and the understanding students have of health.

---

[3] *Health Is Academic: A Guide to Coordinated School Health Programs.* Edited by Eva Marx, Daphne Northrop, and Susan Frelick Wooley. New York: Teachers College Press, 1998; *Schools and Health: Our Nation's Investment.* Edited by Diane Allensworth and others. Washington, D.C.: National Academy Press, 1997.

Other documents have used the terms *comprehensive health education, comprehensive school health education,* or *comprehensive school health instruction* to describe health education. To avoid confusion and simplify terms, this document uses the term *health education.* However, that choice should not be seen as an attempt to undermine the purpose of addressing all nine content areas and all four unifying ideas.

This edition of the *Health Framework* can be used to support the positive health behaviors of children. The achievement of optimal health, positive health behaviors, and health literacy is a collaborative, supportive effort. Health and learning are interdependent, and a quality health education curriculum imbedded in a coordinated school health program is essential for the accomplishment of all the goals of education.

Schools and Health

The report *Schools and Health: Our Nation's Investment* is noteworthy for its emphasis on scientific research and empirically based findings.[4] In 1994 the Institute of Medicine, a division of the National Academy of Sciences, convened a committee of national experts on school health to carry out a major study of comprehensive school health programs in kindergarten through grade twelve. The committee had several specific charges:

- Develop a framework for determining the desirable and feasible health outcomes, including mental, emotional, and social health, of comprehensive school health programs.
- Examine the relationship between health outcomes and education outcomes.
- Consider which factors are necessary in the school setting in order to optimize those outcomes.
- Appraise existing data on effectiveness, including cost effectiveness, of comprehensive school health programs and identify possible additional strategies for evaluating the effectiveness of those programs.
- Recommend mechanisms for wider implementation of health programs that have proven to be effective.

A series of meetings brought committee members together with numerous other experts on school health to develop position papers addressing each of the key focus areas, after which the committee published its findings and recommendations in *Schools and Health.*

One of the report's most important conclusions is that "the period prior to high school is the most crucial for shaping attitudes and behaviors. By the time students reach high school, many are already engaging in risky behaviors or

---

[4] See note 3.

may at least have formed accepting attitudes toward these behaviors."[5] Given that premise, *Schools and Health* provides a platform and a research base on which to build effective school health programs for the future. The report makes the following recommendations:

- All students should receive sequential, age-appropriate health education every year during the elementary and middle or junior high grades and a minimum of a one-semester health education course at the secondary level.
- All elementary teachers should receive substantive preparation in health education content and methodology during their preservice college training.
- School health services should be formally planned, and the quality of services should be continuously monitored as an integral part of the community public health and primary care systems.
- Research should be conducted on school-based services, particularly on the organization, management, efficacy, and cost-effectiveness of extended services.
- Confidentiality of health records should be given high priority by the school, and confidential records should be handled in a manner similar to the way in which health records are handled in nonschool health care settings.
- Established sources of funding for school health services should continue from both public health and education funds, and new approaches to funding should be developed.
- Federal leadership for coordinated school health programs should be revitalized by reaffirming the mission of the federal Interagency Committee on School Health (ICSH) and related leadership organizations.
- An official state interagency coordinating council for school health should be established in each state to integrate the diverse elements of coordinated school health systems.
- Every school district should establish a formal organization with broad representation to function as a coordinating council for school health.
- Individual schools should establish a school health committee and appoint a school health coordinator to oversee the school health program.
- The training and use of competent, properly prepared personnel should be expanded to implement quality coordinated school health programs.
- An active research agenda on coordinated school health programs should be pursued and a major research effort launched to establish model programs and studies.
- Further study should be carried out in each of the components of coordinated school health programming.

---

[5] *Schools and Health*, p. 140.

Schools and Health is based on the assumption that education and health are closely linked and that schools have the potential to become an important element in addressing the health needs of children and youths. The report also acknowledges that much work needs to be done and that coordinated school health programs and systems exist more as a concept than as a reality. The purpose of the report is to provide the research, analysis, and recommendations to bring about lasting change and move the field forward significantly.

Health Is Academic provides documentation on the critical link between health and learning. It begins with this quote from the National Commission on the Role of the School and the Community in Improving Adolescent Health: "Efforts to improve school performance that ignore health are ill-conceived, as are health improvement efforts that ignore education."[6]

Many school leaders indicate that their efforts to coordinate health programs result in improved attendance, less smoking among students and staff, lower rates of teen pregnancy, increased participation in physical fitness activities, and healthier dietary choices. School leaders have found that greater use of school health and counseling services decreases disciplinary problems and can delay the onset of health-risk behaviors that jeopardize students' health and academic achievement.

Both *Schools and Health* and *Health Is Academic* substantiate the need for a coordinated approach to school health programs and a framework with fundamental guidelines on how to implement a coordinated program model through school, parent, and community collaboration.

Unifying Ideas of Health Literacy

Health-literate individuals develop a growing mastery of knowledge, skills, and behaviors in four key areas critical to healthy living:

- *Acceptance of personal responsibility for lifelong health.* Health-literate individuals acknowledge that they have some control over their health, incorporate health-related knowledge into everyday behavior, and make a lifelong commitment to healthy living.

- *Respect for and promotion of the health of others.* Health-literate individuals understand and acknowledge the effects of personal behavior on the health and well-being of others. In addition, they understand the influence that people have on the environment and the way in which elements within the environment affect the health of groups and individuals. They translate this understanding into concern for the health of others in the family, school, peer group, and community.

For the first time in recent history, the next generation of Californians may not be as well off as the one which preceded it.

—*Children Now,
1992 Annual Report:
Saving the Dream*

---

[6] *Health Is Academic,* p. 1.

- *An understanding of the process of growth and development.* Health-literate individuals understand and acknowledge the aspects of physical, mental, emotional, and social growth and development common to all people as well as those aspects that are unique to individuals. They respect the dignity of all individuals and recognize that people continue to develop throughout their lives.

- *Informed use of health-related information, products, and services.* Health-literate individuals select and use available health-related information, products, and services carefully and wisely. Being health literate involves the ability to think critically about health-related information and be a selective consumer of health-related services and products.

The four unifying ideas of health literacy are central themes throughout this framework and are reiterated and reinforced in a variety of contexts.

The School's Role in Promoting Children's Health

Growing numbers of children are coming to school with a variety of health-related problems that make successful learning difficult or impossible, and many children in school routinely participate in behaviors that endanger their health. Many of the most serious health problems in our society affect the school-age population. A Children's Defense Fund report concluded that because of declining access to health services, children under eighteen years of age are at increasing risk of contracting infectious diseases and developing physical and mental disabilities. The report also pointed to the rising incidence of such preventable childhood diseases as measles, mumps, and rubella.[7] A national study on adolescents conducted by the U.S. Centers for Disease Control and Prevention (CDC) found alarming levels of the use of alcohol and other drugs, weapon-carrying among high school students, early sexual activity, and suicide. CDC has determined that the most detrimental health-risk behaviors practiced by young people fall into six categories: (1) behaviors that result in unintentional or intentional injuries; (2) use of alcohol and other drugs; (3) sexual behaviors that result in HIV infection, other sexually transmitted diseases, or unintended pregnancy; (4) use of tobacco; (5) unhealthy diet; and (6) reduced physical activity.[8]

Trends in California are consistent with disturbing national findings. Although California's teen birth rate has declined in recent years, it remains higher than the teen birth rate in many other states. The percentage of incarcerated juveniles is also high. Many juveniles are confined, directly or indirectly,

School programs need to recognize the bidirectional connection between health and education. Children must be healthy in order to be educated and children must be educated in order to stay healthy.

—Public Health Reports

---

[7] *The Health of America's Children.* Washington, D.C.: Children's Defense Fund, 1992.

[8] *Chronic Disease and Health Promotion: Reprints from the MMWR 1990-1991 Youth Risk Behavior Surveillance System.* Atlanta: Centers for Disease Control and Prevention, n.d.

because of their use of alcohol or other drugs or because of their possession or use of weapons. Further, California's children tend to be physically unfit. They have higher percentages of body fat, are less physically active, and score lower on objective measures of physical fitness than in the past. Injuries, intentional or unintentional, which are the leading cause of death and disability among children and youths in California, have had an enormous impact. On average eight children in California die from injuries every day, and many more are seriously disabled.

An article appearing in *Public Health Reports* emphasizes the combined roles of the education and health sectors in promoting lifelong good health.[9] The Healthy Kids, Healthy California Initiative, launched by the California Department of Education in 1989, and the Healthy Start Initiative (Senate Bill 620/1991) support the development of a positive, health-oriented school climate that recognizes health as being intimately linked to learning.

An emphasis on health is consistent with the goals for school reform in California. The major policy and planning documents that will influence California's schools for many years to come acknowledge that good health is basic to academic success.[10] A common theme is the need for schools to take an active role in developing and promoting the physical, mental, emotional, and social health of students. The documents also call for students to be engaged in meaningful work. Because health is relevant to students, health-related tasks can be used to capture student interest and enhance development of knowledge and skills in other curriculum areas.

Working with families and the community, schools have a unique opportunity to influence the health of children positively. In the past many schools resisted allocating resources to health beyond the bare minimum because evidence of its benefits was insufficient. Health seemed to have little relevance to day-to-day learning. Today, however, the benefits of health education and coordinated school health approaches are clear. Many studies have found that school-based programs have brought about positive changes in a wide range of health-related behaviors among children, such as decision making and the ability to resist negative influences.[11] Researchers have found that instruction combining scientifically based information about health issues and continual reinforcement of positive health behaviors can also be effective.

---

[9] A. C. Novello and others, "Healthy Children Ready to Learn: An Essential Collaboration Between Health and Education," *Public Health Reports*, Vol. 107, No. 1 (1992), 3–14.

[10] See California Department of Education publications *Here They Come: Ready or Not! Report of the School Readiness Task Force*, 1988; *It's Elementary! Elementary Grades Task Force Report*, 1992; *Caught in the Middle: Educational Reform for Young Adolescents in California Public Schools*, 1987; *Second to None: A Vision of the New California High School*, 1992.

[11] D. Kirby and others, "Reducing the Risk: Impact of a New Curriculum on Sexual Risk-Taking," *Journal of School Health*, Vol. 23, No. 6 (1991), 253–63. See also J. R. Seffrin, "The Comprehensive School Health Curriculum: Closing the Gap Between State-of-the-Art and State-of-the-Practice," *Journal of School Health*, Vol. 60, No. 4 (1990), 151–56.

Through education and comprehensive prevention strategies developed and implemented with parent involvement and education, schools can influence health behaviors significantly. They can state explicitly that certain behaviors are unhealthy but that other behaviors will enhance health and well-being. For example, schools can state that (1) violent behavior and actions that demean others are not acceptable; (2) alcohol, tobacco, and other drugs are not healthy and should not be used by children and youths; (3) sexual activity is not appropriate for young people; (4) safety practices should be followed and protective equipment and devices, such as seat belts and helmets, should be used; and (5) excessive consumption of fat and insufficient physical activity are not healthy, but healthy food choices and physical activity can enhance health. Schools can teach and model healthy choices and empower young people to take responsibility for their own health and well-being.

Given the needs of today's children and the potential of schools to address children's health issues, schools must make health a priority in the curriculum and the overall school program. Because basic patterns of healthy living are formed in childhood and adolescence, schools, working in partnership with families and communities, are an ideal place to promote healthy attitudes and behaviors.

Collaboration to Benefit the Whole Child

The health of children and their success in school are intimately linked.[12] Increasingly, the value and importance of educating the whole child, including focusing on children's health, is being supported by empirical studies. Inadequate nutrition and a wide range of negative and self-destructive behaviors, such as the use of alcohol, tobacco, and other drugs, have been linked to poor school performance. The converse is also true; that is, children who are helped to accept responsibility for their health are more likely to succeed in school and to become healthier, more responsible, and more successful adults. Schools are collaborating with parents and the community to address problems and behaviors that influence school performance. That approach is central to *Not Schools Alone*, which charts the course for alcohol, tobacco, and other drug education and prevention programs in California schools.[13]

Not Schools Alone emphasizes the importance of the school and the community in influencing children's health. Children and adolescents are more likely to practice healthy behaviors when those behaviors are broadly supported at school, at home, and in the community. A variety of *risk factors* influence whether or

School systems are not responsible for meeting every need of their students. But where the need directly affects learning, the school must meet the challenge. So it is with health.

—*Turning Points: Preparing American Youth for the 21st Century*

---

[12] *School Health: Helping Children Learn.* Alexandria, Va.: National School Boards Association, 1991, pp. 1–5. See also *Promoting Health Education in Schools: A Critical Issues Report.* Arlington, Va.: American Association of School Administrators, 1985, pp. 7–9.

[13] *Not Schools Alone: Guidelines for Schools and Communities to Prevent the Use of Tobacco, Alcohol, and Other Drugs Among Children and Youth.* Sacramento: California Department of Education, 1991.

For health education to
be made meaningful,
systems must be in place
that support effective
health education and
make health an important
priority in the school.

not a child will be healthy and will maintain a commitment to health. The school, the home, the community, and the peer group are four major areas of a child's life in which these risk factors may be found. The risk factors include, among others, economic deprivation, neighborhood disintegration, poor family-management practices, peers who use alcohol and other drugs, low expectations for children's success, and academic failure. Although some risk factors are far beyond a school's control, others can be addressed directly and effectively through health education supported by collaborative efforts that include parents, the school, and the community.

Balancing, buffering, and reducing risk in children's lives are *protective factors*. They include having opportunities to practice health-related skills, such as decision-making or refusal skills; knowing that clearly defined expectations and norms exist for appropriate behavior at school and at home; experiencing positive bonding to the family, the school, peers, and the community; and receiving recognition for participation in positive activities and personal accomplishments. These protective factors lead to the development of a sense of personal competence and resiliency. Together, schools, families, and the community can work to strengthen the protective factors and build resiliency. The physical, emotional, and social benefits of such collaborative efforts can be significant.

The Benefits of Prevention

Promoting children's health can be highly cost-effective for schools and communities; neglecting it can mean spiraling costs for health care. As the cost of health care continues to increase, disease prevention, health promotion, and access to services are assuming greater importance in the public health agenda.

Recent increases in the incidence of several easily preventable diseases, such as measles and mumps, have underscored the cost-effectiveness of a prevention-oriented approach. For example, a single dose of vaccine against measles, mumps, and rubella costs approximately $25. But the cost of not being vaccinated can be staggering. Complications from measles can result in death or blindness, mumps can leave males sterile, and rubella infection in pregnant women can seriously compromise their pregnancies. Clearly, the cost of prevention is far less than the cost to treat those diseases and their complications.

Prevention and collaboration to ensure adequate access to services while avoiding duplication of services have become fundamental components of health policy and health-care reform nationally and statewide. One indication of those trends is the movement toward school-linked services, such as after-school child-care and recreation programs.

For example, California's Healthy Start Initiative (Senate Bill 620/1991) provides funds for schools and community public and private organizations to work together to provide a system of comprehensive, integrated health, psychosocial, and educational services. The school-linked services initiative promotes the reconfiguration of existing community resources. A center at or near the school site serves as the gateway for a continuum of services (such as primary health care, mental-health services, academic support, counseling, parenting education, nutrition services, health education, youth development, or substance-abuse prevention) for students and families who need assistance.

Some services are offered on site. Others are offered through referral from the center's family advocate to a provider in the community. Services are family-focused and prevention- and result-oriented. School-linked services help ensure that existing community resources are used effectively by individuals and families who need assistance. Ongoing collaboration and consultation among school personnel, parents, and service providers result in more efficient and supportive delivery of services. Teachers are able to refer families to needed assistance and community agency staff can target services to families who want help. Together, the school, the school-linked service providers, and the family provide consistent efforts to support the student's success at school. (See Appendix B for an example of school-linked services.)

Structures for a Coordinated School Health System

Preventing health problems, promoting health literacy, and supporting students' success at school through a comprehensive, collaborative approach may involve significant changes at some schools. However, working with families and the community, schools can establish an effective system for preventing health problems and promoting health literacy.

This framework envisions a coordinated school health system based on the assumption, strongly supported by research and practice, that the teaching of health information alone is insufficient for children and youths to achieve health literacy. Effective health education must combine scientifically based information with approaches that develop positive health attitudes and behaviors and incorporate a wide range of learning styles, activities, and teaching strategies. It engages children on many different levels to develop knowledge, skills, attitudes, and behaviors that will make health education not the presentation of a set of facts to be studied, memorized, and quickly forgotten but a meaningful part of children's lives. In addition, it relates health information to a variety of disciplines and learning situations.

For health education to be made meaningful, systems must be in place that support effective health education and make health an important priority in the school. The school's approach must be well planned, must be coherent, must be implemented consistently, and must be supported by all adults in the school. All the components of the school's program must be mutually supportive and

The school's approach must be well planned, must be coherent, must be implemented consistently, and must be supported by all adults in the school. All the components of the school's program must be mutually supportive and consistent with the overall goal of promoting and enhancing children's health literacy.

consistent with the overall goal of promoting and enhancing children's health literacy.

This schoolwide approach is referred to in this framework as a *coordinated school health system* with eight components:[14]

- Health Education
- Physical Education
- Nutrition Services
- Health Services
- Psychological and Counseling Services
- Safe and Healthy School Environment
- Health Promotion for Staff
- Parent and Community Involvement

These eight components work together to develop and reinforce health-related knowledge, skills, attitudes, and behaviors and make health an important priority at the school. The components are linked in a mutually supportive, cooperative system focusing on children's health issues and the development of health literacy. Each of the eight components is a critical link in the overall support system for school health and is integrally related to the other components. Some of the components focus on education, others on services, and still others on the school environment. When they are planned and implemented in a supportive and consistent manner, the eight components achieve far more in promoting health literacy than is possible without a coherent, integrated system. The entire support system is shown in figure 1.

- *Health education and physical education* focus on helping students gain the knowledge, skills, and behaviors needed for health literacy and on engendering the attitudes they also need for lifelong healthy behaviors. Health education is the primary focus of this framework. Physical education taught within the context of a coordinated school health system is the subject of its own framework. Readers seeking detailed information about the design of exemplary physical education curriculum should consult the *Physical Education Framework*.

- *Health services, nutrition services, and psychological and counseling services* reinforce the knowledge, skills, and behaviors taught in health education and physical education; help families support and promote students' health; and provide students with opportunities to practice healthy behaviors. For example, school nutrition services support healthy growth and development by providing nutritious foods to students. School nutrition services also offer students opportunities to apply knowledge

---

[14] The model of a coordinated school health system described in this framework was most recently presented in the Healthy Kids, Healthy California Initiative. For information about the initiative, contact the Safe and Healthy Kids Program Office, California Department of Education, 1430 N Street, Sacramento (mailing address: P.O. Box 944272, Sacramento, CA 94244-2720); telephone 916-319-0920.

Fig. 1. A Coordinated School Health System

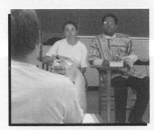
Health Education

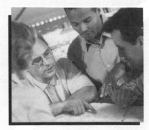
Parent and Community Involvement

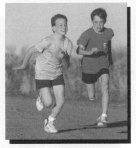
Physical Education

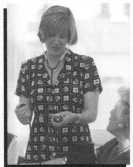
Health Promotion for Staff

Eight Components of a Coordinated School Health System

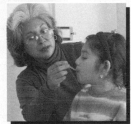
Health Services

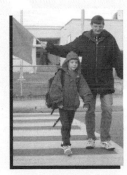
Safe and Healthy School Environment

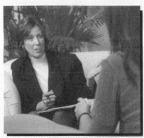
Psychological and Counseling Services

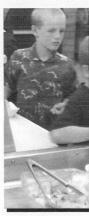
Nutrition Services

of nutrition learned in the classroom to their selection of nutritious foods at school.

Health services, including early and periodic health screenings, such as examinations of vision and hearing, provided at or near the school site offer students access to vital health care that is often not available to them from any other source. Psychological and counseling services provided at or near the school site offer students assistance and support in making healthy decisions, coping with crises, and resolving or managing problems that might influence success at school. When provided in the context of a coordinated school health system, these types of services can also help students and their families find the support they need in a coordinated and effective manner.

- *Safe and healthy school environment, health promotion for staff, and parent and community involvement* all support and reinforce the school's commitment to the development of health literacy. A safe and healthy school environment ensures that students and adults at the school site are physically safe and that the school environment supports health literacy and successful learning. Health promotion for staff empowers teachers and other staff members to make a commitment to lifelong healthy behaviors and model those behaviors for students. In addition, parent and community involvement brings parents, the community, and the school together to develop and support health literacy. As a result the school views itself as an integral part of the community and works in partnership with parents to promote the success of students.

Parents and the community are involved in a variety of roles in the school, ranging from occasional volunteering to active, meaningful leadership on school committees. Parent and community involvement, health promotion for staff, and a safe and healthy school environment all contribute to developing a schoolwide commitment to health. Each of these components should be developed and supported as a necessary part of the coordinated school health system. Together, the components of a coordinated school health system empower students to develop and apply knowledge and skills leading to healthy choices and lifelong good health. This system provides the school and community with a sound approach for preventing health problems when possible and dealing with them in a systematic way when they do occur. When a well-designed curriculum and a supporting structure are available, the goal of health literacy for all children is realistic and achievable.

When a well-designed curriculum and a supporting structure are available, the goal of health literacy for all children is realistic and achievable.

Parents as Providers and Decision Makers

Parents and guardians should be closely involved in the design and implementation of efforts to support children's health from the very beginning of the process. This involvement should go well beyond token participation.

Why is it important to involve parents? First, it helps to keep the planning and implementation of the coordinated school health system on the right track. As experts on their children and on their own communities, parents can ensure that schools address the issues that families and communities perceive as relevant. Second, active participation is in itself an intervention for the individual parents who get involved. Providing individuals with opportunities to be connected, to grow and develop, and to give back to their community allows them to see new possibilities for themselves. Third, involving parents builds the community's capacity for self-sufficiency. Community members learn to do for themselves and each other, rather than wait for an outside person or group to provide for them or to lead them. Fourth, community parents can bring valuable assets to family outreach work, including a knowledge of different community cultures and languages, an ability, as peers, to build close and trusting relationships quickly, and an ability to identify unique solutions to problems that professionals might not see.

Therefore, schools should involve parents in developing and providing support activities, such as organizing transportation, following up with tardy children in the neighborhood each morning, overseeing an after-school study club, organizing parent support groups on various topics, fund-raising for small projects, and so on. Schools may also consider involving parents in more paraprofessional types of support, such as individual peer counseling or case management. When parents will be filling paraprofessional roles, the school must provide parents with the necessary training in maintaining confidentiality, keeping records, conducting interviews, and so forth.

Parents and guardians should also be key decision makers on policy issues and should be represented in sufficient numbers to have an impact. Parents should be involved in all decisions that will affect them, especially on such matters as which services are to be offered to families and how services should be adapted to make them culturally meaningful.

Positive Youth Development, Asset Development, and Resiliency

The developmental assets that link individual resiliency with positive health behavior are an increasingly important part of a coordinated school health system. The importance of using related data to determine needs, develop plans, and evaluate the components of coordinated school health programs is highlighted in this section.

The concept of positive youth development, often in association with the development of *resiliency* and developmental *assets* among youths, has gained wide attention and support among proponents of coordinated school health programs. To a great extent, that support has been brought about by a growing body of psychological and sociological research on youth development that links individual resiliency and developmental assets with health promotion and disease prevention.

The document *Getting Results, Update 1: Positive Youth Development: Research, Commentary, and Action* focuses entirely on research, commentary, and specific programs and activities related to positive youth development.[15] This document, which contains numerous references to additional sources of information on the topic, is an essential starting point and will lead to further readings. It also contains an optional module on resilience assessment from the *California Healthy Kids Survey.*

Before schools proceed in developing a school health program, it is important to establish definitions of the terms that are most often encountered in the promotion of health and prevention of disease among youths:

Youth development. An approach that helps youths build strong relationships with others, learn new skills, and give back to the community

Resiliency. The ability to bounce back in the face of adversity; the ability to weather the effects of stress, insult, and injury (This area of research and practice is grounded in environmental and psychological factors that help children transcend adversity.)

Developmental assets. The building blocks of human development, such as family support, creative activities, and achievement motivation, that promote health and protect young people from risk-taking behaviors

External protective factors. Peer, family, school, and community influences on youths' attitudes, perceptions, and behaviors; external supports and opportunities, such as caring relationships, high expectations, and opportunities to participate and contribute

---

[15] *Getting Results, Update 1: Positive Youth Development: Research, Commentary, and Action.* Sacramento: California Department of Education, 1999.

Internal protective factors. Individual attitudes, perceptions, and behaviors (e.g., self-efficacy, positive beliefs about self)

Pioneering research on resiliency was done by the psychologist Emmy Werner, who for more than three decades studied the development of 700 children born on the Hawaiian island of Kauai. As described in Bonnie Benard's summary of a report by Werner and fellow psychologist Ruth S. Smith, approximately one-third of the children were at significant risk of a variety of personal and health problems. Yet when these high-risk children were studied at the age of eighteen, about one-third were "doing well in getting along with parents and peers, doing fine in school, avoiding serious trouble, and having good mental health."[16] A follow-up study of the same cohort at age thirty-two found that some two-thirds of the adolescents who were at high risk at age eighteen had become healthy, competent, caring, successful adults.[17]

An analysis of those findings led Werner and Smith to theorize that, despite stressful childhood environments that place children at high risk of numerous personal and health-related problems, many youths develop protective factors that help them to function successfully and effectively throughout their lives. The main protective factors, according to this research, are as follows:

- The development of social skills that enable people to reach out to family members and others for support
- The presence of a committed caregiver, particularly during the first year of life
- A broad community support system[18]

As interest in the concept of protective factors has grown, health educators and youth advocates have increasingly questioned the major assumptions on which youth-focused health promotion and disease prevention programs traditionally have been based. The dominant model, observes Peter L. Benson, a leading developmental assets researcher with the independent Search Institute, focuses on the concept of deficit reduction: "naming, counting, and reducing the negative;" that is, reducing risks to young people's health and well-being.[19] The converse is a focus on positive aspects of young people's development—protective factors and developmental assets that help young people to function

---

[16] Bonnie Benard, "Resiliency Study," in *Getting Results, Part I: California Action Guide to Creating Safe and Drug-Free Schools and Communities.* Sacramento: California Department of Education, 1998, p. 136, citing Emmy E. Werner and Ruth S. Smith, *Vulnerable but Invincible: A Longitudinal Study of Resilient Children and Youth.* New York: Adams, Bannister, and Cox, 1989.

[17] Bonnie Benard, citing Emmy E. Werner and Ruth S. Smith, *Overcoming the Odds: High-Risk Children from Birth to Adulthood.* New York: Cornell University Press, 1992.

[18] Ibid.

[19] Peter L. Benson, "Promoting Positive Human Development: The Power of Schools," in *Getting Results, Update 1,* p. 14.

and grow in ways that lead to personal success, competence, effectiveness, health, and well-being. Researcher Michael D. Resnick notes that a major assumption of the positive youth development approach is that "young people are resources to be treasured and developed, not problems to be solved."[20]

The Search Institute is an independent, nonprofit, nonsectarian organization whose mission is to advance the well-being of adolescents and children by generating knowledge and promoting the application of that knowledge. The institute's research has resulted in the identification of 40 developmental assets.

Developmental Assets Identified by the Search Institute

In 1990 the Search Institute compiled 40 developmental assets, relying on research on child and adolescent development, risk prevention, and resiliency. Research surveys of more than one million sixth graders and twelfth graders show that youths who experience these assets are more likely to make healthy choices and avoid a wide range of high-risk behaviors than are youths who do not experience these assets, which are described as follows:

EXTERNAL ASSETS

Support

1. **Family support**—Family life provides high levels of love and support.
2. **Positive family communication**—Young person and her or his parent(s) communicate positively, and young person is willing to seek advice and counsel from parent(s).
3. **Other adult relationships**—Young person receives support from three or more non-parent adults.
4. **Caring neighborhood**—Young person experiences caring neighbors.
5. **Caring school climate**—School provides a caring, encouraging environment.
6. **Parent involvement in schooling**—Parent(s) are actively involved in helping young person succeed in school.

Empowerment

7. **Community that values youths**—Young person perceives that adults in the community value youths.

Developmental Assets reprinted with permission from the Search Institute, Minneapolis, Minn. © Search Institute, 1996. *http://www.search-institute.org.*

---

[20] Michael D. Resnick, "Resiliency, Protective Factors, and Connections That Count in the Lives of Adolescents," in *Getting Results, Update 1*, p. 29, citing Milbrey W. McLaughlin and others, *Urban Sanctuaries: Neighborhood Organizations in the Lives and Futures of Inner-City Youth.* San Francisco: Jossey-Bass, Inc., 1994.

8. **Youths as resources**—Young people are given useful roles in the community.

9. **Service to others**—Young person serves in the community one hour or more per week.

10. **Safety**—Young person feels safe at home, at school, and in the neighborhood.

Boundaries and Expectations

11. **Family boundaries**—Family has clear rules and consequences and monitors the young person's whereabouts.

12. **School boundaries**—School provides clear rules and consequences.

13. **Neighborhood boundaries**—Neighbors take responsibility for monitoring young people's behavior.

14. **Adult role models**—Parent(s) and other adults model positive, responsible behavior.

15. **Positive peer influence**—Young person's best friends model responsible behavior.

16. **High expectations**—Both parent(s) and teachers encourage the young person to do well.

Constructive Use of Time

17. **Creative activities**—Young person spends three or more hours per week in lessons or practice in music, theater, or other arts.

18. **Youth programs**—Young person spends three or more hours per week in sports, clubs, or organizations at school and/or in the community.

19. **Religious community**—Young person spends one or more hours per week in activities in a religious institution.

20. **Time at home**—Young person is out with friends "with nothing special to do" two or fewer nights per week.

INTERNAL ASSETS

Commitment to Learning

21. **Achievement motivation**—Young person is motivated to do well in school.

22. **School engagement**—Young person is actively engaged in learning.

23. **Homework**—Young person reports doing at least one hour of homework every school day.

24. **Bonding to school**—Young person cares about her or his school.

25. **Reading for pleasure**—Young person reads for pleasure three or more hours per week.

Positive Values

26.   **Caring**—Young person places high value on helping other people.
27.   **Equality and social justice**—Young person places high value on promoting equality and reducing hunger and poverty.
28.   **Integrity**—Young person acts on convictions and stands up for her or his beliefs.
29.   **Honesty**—Young person "tells the truth even when it is not easy."
30.   **Responsibility**—Young person accepts and takes personal responsibility.
31.   **Restraint**—Young person believes it is important not to be sexually active or to use alcohol or other drugs.

Social Competencies

32.   **Planning and decision making**—Young person knows how to plan ahead and make choices.
33.   **Interpersonal competence**—Young person has empathy, sensitivity, and friendship skills.
34.   **Cultural competence**—Young person has knowledge of and comfort with people of different cultural/racial/ethnic backgrounds.
35.   **Resistance skills**—Young person can resist negative peer pressure and dangerous situations.
36.   **Peaceful conflict resolution**—Young person seeks to resolve conflict nonviolently.

Positive Identity

37.   **Personal power**—Young person feels she or he has control over "things that happen to me."
38.   **Self-esteem**—Young person reports having a high self-esteem.
39.   **Sense of purpose**—Young person reports, "my life has purpose."
40.   **Positive view of personal future**—Young person is optimistic about her or his future.

Implementation of Youth Development

Despite significant new research on the importance of resiliency and developmental assets, the concept of positive youth development cannot be reduced to a simple curriculum or program. As noted by Benson, "There are no magic potions or quick fixes that steer lives toward success, productivity, and responsibility."[21] Rather, promoting resiliency among children and youths and emphasizing developmental assets need to be part of a schoolwide and communitywide approach to nurturing and fostering healthy, productive young people. Although specific program components and curricula can be

---

[21] Peter L. Benson, p. 15.

helpful in implementing a broad-based health strategy of this kind, implementation should take many different factors into account, including the following action steps suggested in *Getting Results, Update 1:*

- An emphasis on cooperation, pro-social development, and positive relationships among children and youths
- A focus on developing a positive and cooperative school climate
- Program planning and development that involves and empowers children and youths in taking a positive and active role in their schools and communities (e.g., through participation in school and community service programs)
- Peer leadership and peer-helping programs
- Training for school staff in positive youth development concepts and approaches[22]

Use of Evaluation and Survey Data in School Health Programs

Why evaluate school health programs? Schools and communities need data to guide their program decision making and development, to obtain program support and funding, and to demonstrate progress in meeting their program goals. Schools are required increasingly to collect data that objectively assess student achievement and behavior. Schools also are encouraged to set concrete and measurable goals for making improvement. Researchers Sarvela and McDermott indicate that the purpose of evaluation is to improve rather than to prove and that evaluation is the process of sharing accountability, not assigning accountability.[23] Other research finds that the essential function of evaluation should be to collect, analyze, and report valid, credible information that can make a constructive impact on program decision making.[24]

Some Basic Terms

The following basic terms are used in the ensuing discussion of evaluation and survey data:

Data. Facts and figures from which conclusions can be inferred

Evaluation. Systematic collection of valid, credible information on the operation of a program, the effects of the program, other questions of interest, or a combination of such information

---

[22] "Research into Action: Action Steps for Schools," in *Getting Results, Update 1,* pp. 55–61.

[23] Paul D. Sarvela and Robert J. McDermott, *Health Education Evaluation and Measurement: A Practitioner's Perspective.* Dubuque, Iowa: Brown and Benchmark, 1993.

[24] Joan L. Herman, Lynn Lyons Morris, and Carol Taylor Fitz-Gibbon, *Evaluator's Handbook.* Newbury Park, Calif.: Sage Publications, 1987.

Evaluation design. A plan that determines the groups or individuals who will participate in an evaluation, the types of data that will be collected, and when the evaluation instruments or means will be administered and by whom

Program. Action taken to cause an effect

Stakeholders. Groups of people who have a direct or indirect interest in evaluation results

Survey. A detailed study made by gathering and analyzing information

Evaluation and Survey Considerations

Many youth health behavior surveys are conducted, and none should be mistaken for an evaluation. Changes in behavior rates, by themselves, do not explain why and how the changes occurred. The changes may not be the effect of a current program, but rather one from prior years that may be showing long-term effects. In any program it is advisable to include an evaluation component. An evaluation may have one of many purposes, such as attainment of program objectives, assessment of strengths and weaknesses, acquisition of data for decision making, or monitoring of standards of performance.

Reliance on health behavior survey measures alone to demonstrate successful health education programs is not advisable because knowledge and skills often are not put into practice. The ultimate goal of health promotion is the practice of positive health behaviors. Those behaviors are preceded by knowledge and skills. It is important to measure these indicators as benchmarks of teaching and learning effectiveness, and the *Health Framework* clearly delineates skill and knowledge expectations at the various grade levels. (Refer to "Resources for Program Planning" and "Health Literacy Assessment" in Chapter 2 for more information on health education assessment strategies.)

In the planning of an evaluation or a survey, several factors should be considered:

- What is the purpose of the data?
- Who are the stakeholders and decision makers who will review the data?
- What kind of data are needed to make decisions or to tailor the evaluation or data presentation to the interests of the identified stakeholders?

At least five different categories of stakeholders and the characteristics of their interests must be considered when planning data collection or evaluation or both:

1. **The organization,** to justify program costs, gain support for programs, satisfy accountability for funding agencies, or determine future program plans
2. **The program administrator,** to bring favorable attention to the program, increase probability for promotion, or gain greater control of the program

3. **The funding agency,** to ensure efficiency, demonstrate program effects, or gain political favor and possibly additional funding

4. **The public,** to ensure that tax dollars are spent efficiently, learn about the benefits/disadvantages of a program, or increase public participation in programs

5. **Program evaluator,** to help support the program's goals, contribute to disciplinary and applied knowledge, or advance professionally

As the research concludes: "Evaluation, in short, is an endeavor which is partly social, partly political, and only partly technical."[25]

Basic Evaluation Models

According to Sarvela and McDermott, most evaluators organize evaluation into two general areas—formative and summative:

- *Formative evaluation* refers to the ongoing process of evaluation while a program is being developed and implemented. The primary goal is to improve the program. For example, a typical formative evaluation question would be whether or not the program's curricular materials match the program's objectives. Sometimes formative evaluations are referred to as process evaluations because they are designed to examine the processes that are taking place while the program is being developed and implemented.

- *Summative evaluation* assesses the degree to which a program has met predetermined objectives or the degree to which the program has been of use to its target population. Summative evaluations most often use quantitative approaches. Quantitative procedures include experimental design and the use of standardized achievement tests or other objective measures.[26]

A good evaluation reference is an essential tool for the health program professional. Several agencies and Web sites that offer guidance on the evaluation process are listed in Additional References and Resources.

Some Cautions About Surveys

Health surveys can bring about controversy, causing concern among officials that the results will make the school or community "look bad." Survey planning should involve parents and community members. Effective use of data begins with the building of community consensus on why the survey is being conducted and how the information will be used. Such involvement will foster allies in the community and among parents, whose contributions to the presentation of the results to the community might be of significant value.

---

[25] Joan L. Herman and others, p. 11.

[26] Paul D. Sarvela and Robert J. McDermott.

Surveys on school violence and high-risk behaviors are not particularly effective when administered only once. The real value of survey data is realized when data are gathered over the course of several years. It is the only way in which trends in the nation, state, school, or district can be discerned. Although comparisons to state and national samples are important, the bottom-line question that must be answered at the local level is "Are we doing better?" Most behaviors do not change dramatically in one year. As a general rule, it is recommended that schools conduct a student health survey every two years in selected student populations.

Parental Consent

All health-risk behavior surveys conducted in schools are confidential and anonymous. They require written parental consent for student participation. Parents must be fully informed about the information requested in the survey, the purpose of the survey, and the intent when the results are published. Student participation in the survey is voluntary, and students may decline to answer any or all of the questions. *Education Code* Section 51513 states, "No test, questionnaire, survey, or examination containing any questions about the pupil's personal beliefs or practices in sex, family life, morality, and religion, or any questions about the pupil's parents' or guardians' beliefs and practices in sex, family life, morality, and religion, shall be administered to any pupil in kindergarten or grades 1 to 12, inclusive, unless the parent or guardian of the pupil is notified in writing that this test, questionnaire, survey, or examination is to be administered and the parent or guardian of the pupil gives written permission for the pupil to take this test, questionnaire, survey, or examination."

Current Data on the Health-Related Behaviors of Young People

The health of young people is linked to the health-related behavior they choose to adopt. According to the Centers for Disease Control and Prevention, a limited number of behaviors contribute markedly to today's major health problems. These behaviors, often established during youth, include:

- Tobacco use
- Unhealthy dietary behaviors
- Inadequate physical activity
- Alcohol and other drug use
- Sexual behaviors that may result in HIV infection, other sexually transmitted diseases, and unintended pregnancies
- Behaviors that may result in intentional injuries (violence and suicide) and unintentional injuries (motor vehicle crashes)

Over the last decade substantial information has been gained about the prevalence of behaviors by young people that put their health at risk. Many sources of survey data exist from which to choose in meeting a variety of program evaluation and planning needs.

Multiple data sources should be used to confirm, enrich, and provide context to an assessment. Comparisons of local, county, state, and national data can help interpret and give meaning to the profile of the student population that is being assessed. The following descriptions of the various types of available survey data are offered to assist in the selection of data sources.

Local Surveys

Support for school programs is often undermined by a lack of local awareness—or even denial—of the extent of youth health risks on campus. Many factors that contribute to health-risk behaviors by youths are also found outside the school setting. Prevention researchers have long recognized the importance of changing the general social environment and norms in order to sustain the impact of school-based programs. Drug use, violence, and other health-risk behaviors are the concern and responsibility of the entire community. Schools and the community must work together to prevent and reduce health-risk behaviors and increase academic achievement among youths.

The *California Healthy Kids Survey* (CHKS) is a comprehensive youth health-risk and resilience data collection system sponsored by the California Department of Education and is available to all local educational agencies (LEAs). The elementary school version of CHKS is an easily customized, self-report youth survey that assesses all major areas of health-related risk behavior and resilience. This low-cost survey support system uses the latest technology to help local agencies collect and use CHKS data to improve prevention and health programs. (See the CHKS Web site at *<http://www.wested.org/hks/>*.)

The secondary school version of CHKS consists of a general core (Module A) and a set of five in-depth, behavior-specific, optional supplementary modules that an LEA can configure to meet local needs and standards. Individual modules assess youth development and resilience (Module B); alcohol- and other drug-use prevention (Module C); tobacco-use prevention (Module D); physical health and nutrition (Module E); and sexual behavior and pregnancy (Module F). A single elementary school instrument provides comparable, developmentally appropriate data focusing on risk and resilience factors.

A growing body of research provides evidence of external and internal factors that protect some adolescents from engagement in a variety of risk behaviors and foster positive developmental outcomes. The CHKS resilience module, developed with the assistance of a national panel of experts, provides a measure of local protective factors and resilience traits or assets. It can help identify the strength of students' external assets in the school, family, community, and peer environments as well as the degree and nature of internal assets among students. It can provide a positive balance to the profile of a community.

State Surveys

The *California Student Survey* (CSS) is a biennial survey sponsored by the Office of the Attorney General since 1985. The survey has now been expanded to a comprehensive health risk survey that covers all of the items in the CHKS general core. CSS is a good source of statewide data representative of all students in California. (See the CSS Web site at *<http://caag.state.ca.us/cvpc/schoolsurvey.htm>*.)

The *California Safe Schools Assessment* provides annual data on the incidents of reported crimes on campus, notably drug use and violence.

National Surveys

The *Youth Risk Behavior Survey* (YRBS) is a biennial national-level survey and is conducted during the even-numbered years. California uses a random procedure to select schools for the state sample. Schools with larger enrollments have a greater chance of being included in the sample. (See the YRBS Web site at *<http://www.cdc.gov/nccdphp/dash/yrbs/index.htm>*.)

Additional Sources

Many other sources of data exist that may be well suited to program planning needs. Examples include the following:

- *California Youth Tobacco Survey,* a statewide telephone tobacco-use survey *<http://www.dhs.cahwnet.gov/tobacco/documents/youthsmoking.pdf>*
- *Fitnessgram,* an annual statewide physical fitness assessment *<http://www.cde.ca.gov/cyfsbranch/lsp/health/pefitnesstest.htm>*
- *Monitoring the Future,* a national survey of alcohol, tobacco, and other drug use *<http://www.monitoringthefuture.org>*
- *School Health Education Profile,* a biennial survey of health education policies and programs in California and the United States *<http://www.cdc.gov/nccdphp/dash/profiles>*

Data Presentation Strategies

The critical principle for the effective presentation of data is to tailor the data to the interests and needs of stakeholders and decision makers. The *California Healthy Kids Survey* is supplemented with a handbook that provides valuable guidance on the collection, organization, use, and presentation of data.

California's Healthy Start Initiative

The Healthy Start initiative, a California state program, was established in 1991 (*Education Code* sections 8800 et seq.) to facilitate partnerships among local educational agencies, families, and communities to benefit children and youths. Healthy Start brings together local school-linked, community-based partnerships to (1) help young people from kindergarten through high school to learn and reach their full potential; and (2) strengthen families and communities.

This initiative takes shape in forms that are as different as are the communities across California in that it builds on the strengths, assets, and needs of each neighborhood. At each local level, the initiative follows a process that includes collaborative decision making, community assessment, prioritization of goals, selection of effective strategies, integration and tracking of initiative components, and evaluation of results. This process is cyclical and continuous; it involves ongoing work to reassess, reevaluate, and reform so that the initiative continues to grow and change along with the community. Healthy Start also provides a process to move communities beyond isolated, separate systems to interconnected teams with children and youths at their center.

The initiative's philosophy is grounded in the belief that educational success, physical health, emotional support, and family and community strength are inseparable. Because the ability to learn well is so important to a successful and happy life, Healthy Start places a special emphasis on improved school performance. The goals of the initiative are as follows:

- Ensure that each child and youth receives the physical, emotional, and intellectual support—in school, at home, and in the community—that he or she needs to learn well.
- Build the capacity of students and parents to be participants, leaders, and decision makers in their schools and communities.
- Help schools and other agencies serving children and families to reorganize, streamline, and integrate their services to provide more effective support to children and their families.

How Healthy Start Works

Because each school-community has its own combination of assets and needs, the "mix" of services and supports varies. Local Healthy Start initiatives may include the following support services:

- Social services providers
- Educators
- Health, mental health, and dental health providers
- Law enforcement personnel

- Employment development counselors
- Recreation, arts, faith, and service organization representatives
- Business representatives
- Student and family peer-support groups

Funding Structures

Healthy Start provides planning grants of up to $50,000, for use over a one- to two-year period, to local educational agencies in collaborative partnerships that demonstrate a readiness to plan for school-integrated support services. Healthy Start also funds operational grants of up to $300,000 and start-up grants of up to $100,000. Healthy Start operational grants are awarded to school-communities that demonstrate an inclusive, collaborative decision-making process that involves students and families in leadership roles; includes a comprehensive community assessment; prioritizes needs and identifies strengths and assets; and includes a plan for integration of effective support services with an emphasis on improved school performance and evaluation to ensure continuous improvement and sustainability. Healthy Start provides 90 percent of the local funding to school-community collaboratives that meet eligibility requirements; for example, elementary schools in which 50 percent of pupils are eligible to receive free and reduced-price meals and middle and high schools in which 35 percent of pupils are eligible to receive free and reduced-price meals. Up to 10 percent of Healthy Start funds can be awarded to schools that qualify under special factors that warrant consideration.

Evaluation Results

Healthy Start evaluation projects are designed by individual grantees. Although individual grantees may choose to collect a variety of data on their programs, educational results are the only data that grantees are required to submit. Each grantee submits an annual report that includes schoolwide data for each school as well as information on the core clients who have been targeted to receive intensive coordinated services. In addition to the educational results, each Healthy Start grantee reports on at least one optional cluster of data that reflects the results each project hopes to achieve for children and families.

Evaluation data were reported for 286 grantees in 1999. The reports included data on almost 7,000 case-managed clients, 75 percent of whom were school-age children and were reported as students most in need. However, because data are not weighted for the size or number of sites, they are not necessarily representative of all Healthy Start core clients statewide. Within these limitations, evaluation results do show that participation in Healthy Start projects correlated with positive impacts.

Among the projects that monitored health indicators of case-managed clients, significant improvements were reported in the following areas:

- Rate of overdue physical exams
- Status of such basic needs as food and shelter
- Rate of substance abuse
- Rate of child abuse

A copy of the complete evaluation report is available from the California Department of Education's Healthy Start Office.

The Healthy Start story is being written in school communities across California. Funding for the Healthy Start initiative (HSI) has grown from an initial level of $19 million in the 1991-92 fiscal year to $39 million in 2001-02. More than 500 operational partnerships at more than 1,200 elementary, middle, and high schools in nearly all of California's 58 counties now have the potential to reach more than one million young people and their families. Participants in Healthy Start around the state live in every kind of community—urban neighborhoods and barrios, rice and cotton fields, resort towns and suburbs, isolated logging towns. Every school and community is different, and every Healthy Start site reflects the unique culture, politics, and economics of its location. What every Healthy Start site shares as part of the coordinated school health "family" is a commitment to making life better for California children, youths, families, and communities. Further information on HSI, including current availability of funds, can be found at the Web site <*http:// www.cde.ca.gov/healthystart*>.

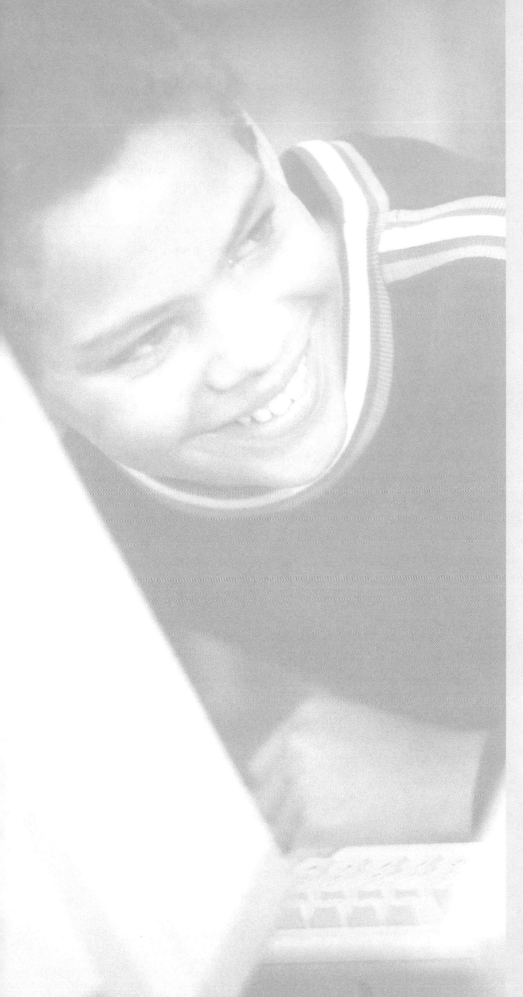

Developing
Health Literacy
in the Classroom
and in the
School

Chapter 2
Developing Health
Literacy in the
Classroom and
in the School

Curriculum reform has
several important
ramifications for
teachers. . . . Teachers
have to redesign their
courses for a higher level
of student work and use
methods that enable
more students to
succeed at this level.

—*Second to None: A Vision
of the New California
High School*

How can schools foster health literacy in all students? This chapter contains suggestions on how schools can deliver quality health education within the context of a coordinated school health system to meet the needs of all students. Although there are many ways to design and implement an effective school health system, this chapter is meant to be a starting point, a guide that schools and school districts can use in creating their own system and overall strategy to promote health literacy. It deals with the elements of successful health education, the effective implementation of a coordinated school health system, research-based school health programs, life skills and positive behaviors, health education planning and development, and the needs of special populations.

Elements of Successful Health Education

To help students develop the knowledge, skills, attitudes, and behaviors needed for a lifelong commitment to health, effective health education:

- *Presents current, accurate content.* All health-related education is based on up-to-date scientific information. It draws on new knowledge about health and maintains a rigorous scientific viewpoint.

- *Recognizes similarities and differences among students.* Effective health education emphasizes the similarities and universal qualities of human beings, helping students see that although differences do exist, many people face similar health-related issues and choices. Regardless of differences in age, culture, disability, ethnic background, gender, primary language, religion, sexual orientation, or socioeconomic background, the students must understand that the knowledge, skills, and behaviors discussed in class apply to all students. Differences should also be discussed, but care should be taken not to emphasize them to the point of divisiveness.

- *Emphasizes not just health-related information but the importance of behavior.* Information alone does not change people's behavior. A lifelong commitment to health results from knowledge, skills, attitudes, and positive behaviors continually repeated and reinforced. Focusing on behavior involves providing students with opportunities to learn, practice, and apply new skills, such as making decisions, refusing negative influences, and accessing health and social service programs to maintain good health. Seen in this way, effective health education does not limit itself to the pages of a textbook but views the school as a safe laboratory for learning, practicing, and reinforcing new behaviors.

- *Is culturally appropriate.* Attitudes, beliefs, and values regarding health-related topics may vary according to the ethnic and cultural makeup of the community. Effective health education should be based on an awareness of the culture and background of students within each classroom and

Chapter 2
Developing Health
Literacy in the
Classroom and
in the School

the influence of culture on the information and skills to be taught. Such an awareness will affect the teaching strategies used and the content of the curriculum. For example, many health education programs teach students how to be assertive and resist negative influences. Yet in some cultures young people are expected to be quiet and obedient, and in other cultures public discussion of certain health-related topics may be considered inappropriate. Whatever the approach, the cultural attitudes and values of the students, their families, and the community must be taken into account.

- *Makes the curriculum accessible.* Not all students learn in the same way, nor are they motivated by the same factors. Therefore, a variety of teaching strategies, both teacher-directed and student-centered, should be used in health education. Activities should provide students with a common experiential base. A variety of grouping strategies allowing students to work individually, in pairs, in small cooperative groups, and in large groups should be used. Instruction should be provided through the primary language and sheltered English whenever possible to make the curriculum accessible to limited-English-proficient (LEP) students. Grouping students to ensure that LEP students have access to bilingual peers, making instructional resources available in the home language, and connecting instruction to students' life experiences will also promote access to the curriculum.

- *Takes advantage of opportunities for active learning.* Every aspect of health education focuses on behaviors or choices, and every topic presents opportunities for engagement and motivation. An effective health education curriculum considers students' needs, appeals to their interests, and capitalizes on those interests in many different ways. It offers abundant opportunities for critical thinking and analysis and remains focused on helping students develop a deep understanding of health literacy. It also provides students with many opportunities to be engaged in creating and constructing what they learn rather than in passively receiving factual information. Students may practice specific skills in the classroom, report on school and community resources for health, and complete meaningful, open-ended homework assignments and large projects that help connect classroom instruction with the home and the community. Classrooms, school cafeterias, nurses' offices, and school-linked community organizations, such as after-school recreation programs or organizations sponsoring community-service projects, should all become laboratories for health-related experiences.

- *Focuses on mental and emotional health throughout.* At one time mental and emotional health was viewed as a separate content area. Increasingly, however, mental and emotional health is considered crucial to an individual's motivation to act on health-related knowledge and use health-related skills. Accordingly, concepts related to mental and emotional

> Effective health education should be based on an awareness of the culture and background of students within each classroom and the influence of culture on the information and skills to be taught.

Chapter 2
Developing Health
Literacy in the
Classroom and
in the School

Through the health education curriculum, students learn strategies for making positive, healthy decisions based on such ethical principles as integrity, courage, responsibility, and commitment.

health are discussed throughout this framework. They are basic to all of health education and are not an independent component that can be covered in a short unit and ignored in the rest of the curriculum.

- *Emphasizes character development.* Health education can promote character development. Through the health education curriculum, students learn strategies for making positive, healthy decisions based on such ethical principles as integrity, courage, responsibility, and commitment. They learn about the importance of consistent choices in all areas of their lives and how those choices affect their health and the health of others. Throughout the health education curriculum, moreover, the development of positive commitments to one's own health and the health of the broader community and society is emphasized.

- *Uses technology to enhance learning.* Technology should be made an integral element of health education. In the classroom students can use technology-based resources to practice skills (e.g., decision making). By using nutrient analysis software, students can assess how the nutritional values of choices for their own meals compare with nutritional standards. They can also develop a personal health profile that tells them where they stand in relation to group norms on a variety of health indicators such as weight and allows them to set and monitor progress toward achieving goals for improvement. In some communities students may have an opportunity to learn to operate analytical instruments used in medical laboratories, in laboratories monitoring environmental conditions, and in clinics and hospitals. Technology can also assist educators. It can help them keep pace with the rapidly changing field of health information; provide network exchanges of instructional programs, resources, services, and research articles; and access resources outside the school and the school district.

- *Focuses on meaning and thinking by connecting concepts in health education with other learning and experiences.* Children learn best when the curriculum is focused on meaning and thinking. Effective health education emphasizes how ideas are connected within the curriculum and with other aspects of the overall school program:

  1. *Connections with other areas of health education.* Effective health education highlights the connections among traditional health topics so that students can explore interrelationships in health. For example, individual growth and development are influenced by nutrition; personal health habits can affect the spread of communicable diseases; and the use of alcohol, tobacco, or other drugs increases the risk of disease and injury.

  2. *Connections with the other components of a coordinated school health system.* Effective health education also links the health curriculum and the other components of a coordinated school health system so that

Chapter 2
Developing Health
Literacy in the
Classroom and
in the School

knowledge and skills learned in the classroom are supported and reinforced throughout the school. For example, the importance of physical fitness in health promotion and disease prevention can be reinforced and enhanced in the physical education class. Further suggestions for connecting the components of a coordinated school health system can be found in Chapter 4.

A note of caution is in order here. Because parental notification is legally mandated before a discussion of human reproductive organs may occur, schools may wish to limit the integration of sex education with other topics.

With these principles of effective health education in place, a foundation can be laid for promoting health literacy and lifelong healthy behaviors. However, health education alone is not enough to promote health literacy in children. Health-related knowledge, skills, attitudes, and behaviors need to be reinforced and supported. The supportive, collaborative structure needed to achieve health literacy can be provided by a coordinated school health system.

Effective Implementation

Having all the components of a coordinated school health system in place will take time and require careful planning. The approaches that have proven successful for program organization and implementation are as follows:

- *Create a common vision.* Although many factors contribute to an effective coordinated school health system, none is more critical than a vision shared by the school and its parents and community. The development of that vision provides a forum for the school and all facets of the community to examine their roles in implementing a coordinated school health system. Once developed, the vision becomes a unifying force for decision making and system development. It should include clearly defined goals and outcomes for all the components of a coordinated school health system.

- *Provide strong administrative support.* The commitment of school and school district leaders is the key to building an effective program. One good way to start is for the school board to develop and adopt a policy clearly stating its commitment and supporting the eight components of a coordinated school health system (see Chapter 1). Specific district policies may already offer guidance on such health matters as dispensing medication, such as that for asthma, providing school nutrition services, or dealing with HIV-infected students. These supporting policies can be reviewed for their consistency in furthering the overall goals and be revised as needed. Because the most effective policies are those that cover

Chapter 2
Developing Health
Literacy in the
Classroom and
in the School

This framework
recommends that the
kindergarten through
grade twelve course of
study in health be
anchored by a full year's
work at the middle
school level and a second
full year's work at the
high school level.

all issues surrounding health and contain enforcement procedures as well,
school districts may choose to combine existing health policies into one
comprehensive policy that contains the vision, goals, and policies and
procedures for implementation and enforcement.

- *Ensure sufficient time for health education.* Because the goal of health
  education is to influence students' lifelong health-related behavior, the
  commitment of a realistic amount of time for health education is essential. Studies have shown that when students receive instruction in health
  education over several years, their health-related behavior is influenced
  positively and significantly. Health education should begin before kindergarten and be continued yearly from kindergarten through grade twelve.
  Several national research studies suggest that significant changes in
  knowledge about health and attitudes toward health seem to occur after
  50 hours of classroom instruction per school year or about one and
  one-half hours per week.[1] This framework recommends that the kindergarten through grade twelve course of study in health be anchored by a
  full year's work at the middle school level and a second full year's work at
  the high school level. Various options exist for including health education
  in the curriculum at those levels, and decisions on how best to offer
  health education should be made locally. What is essential is that adequate amounts of time be allocated for such instruction.

- *Encourage broad-based involvement.* Broad-based involvement is crucial to
  developing and maintaining articulated kindergarten through grade
  twelve health education and instituting a coordinated school health
  system. Many individuals can be involved in a schoolwide effort. Effective
  strategies for creating involvement include the following:

  1. *Forming a school-site health team or health committee.* This group can
     have responsibility for guiding the process, including planning,
     coordinating parent and community involvement, developing
     curriculum, and implementing program components consistently.
     Membership should be representative of the entire school: classroom
     teachers; teachers of health education, physical education, home
     economics, science, and special education; school nurses; counselors;
     school nutrition services personnel; categorical program staff; admin-
     istrators; others at the school site; parents; and community members.
     School-linked service providers, such as social workers, child-care
     providers, recreation specialists, probation officers, and others, may
     also be included.

---

[1] D. Connell and others, "Summary of Findings of the School Health Education Evaluation: Health Promotion Effectiveness, Implementation, and Costs," *Journal of School Health*, Vol. 55, No. 8 (1985), 316–21.

Chapter 2
Developing Health
Literacy in the
Classroom and
in the School

2. *Fostering parent and community involvement.* Parent and community involvement is discussed in more detail in Chapter 4 as one component of a coordinated school health system. However, it is important to note here that strong ties to the community will enhance the school's efforts to promote health literacy. The process of developing a consensus about community needs and wants regarding a coordinated school health system should be continuing, open, and responsive.

3. *Providing mechanisms for effective coordination, collaboration, and communication.* Designating a staff member to coordinate activities and facilitate communication among the various participants helps ensure that these critical activities are handled effectively. The roles and responsibilities of a coordinator might include working with the on-site team and others to assess the school's health education curriculum; providing or arranging for in-service training of staff on health-related issues; maintaining continuing and open communication among school staff; working with the appropriate staff to plan and implement connections between health education and other curriculum areas; organizing meetings to share information with parents and community members; writing grant proposals; monitoring the progress of the overall program; establishing clear and appropriate lines of referral between the school, parents, and community agencies; and maintaining a dialogue with county-level groups involved with services for children and youths.

- *Identify resources for program support.* Many communities are able to provide a variety of resources for a coordinated school health system. Some of these resources (e.g., targeted funding, after-school activities, and staff who can assist with program implementation) are a response to local needs, such as gang activity or a high incidence of drug use. The organizers and coordinators of school-based programs should look to community health and human-service providers for available resources and find ways to create linkages between those resources and the school.

Such linkages can enhance an effective coordinated school health system. Only through the collaborative efforts of school personnel, parents, and community agencies and representatives will most schools be able to assist students and their families in obtaining needed health, mental health, social, and other support services, ranging from basic food, clothing, and housing programs to child-care and recreational programs. These community linkages can also enrich health education by offering real-life experiences to students through health-related issues, practices, and programs.

What makes the difference in a healthy school is that all the people who can have an impact on children's health—administrators, teachers, physical educators, nurses, counselors, support staff, food services staff, family members, community service providers, law enforcement representatives—take time to sit down together and talk about how they can work cooperatively and collaboratively to make the most of the resources available to them.

—*Toward Healthy Schools: The Future Is Now*

Chapter 2
Developing Health
Literacy in the
Classroom and
in the School

Project TEACH
(Teacher Education to
Achieve Comprehensive
Health), funded by the
California Department of
Education and College
Health 2000, was
designed to improve
preservice teacher
training in health
education.
(See Appendix B.)

The entire staff [and
parents] should be
offered training in the
philosophy of the
coordinated school
health system and their
roles in helping students
develop lifelong healthy
behaviors.

- *Provide adequate training.* Different kinds of training and different approaches for diverse audiences will be needed as the school's coordinated school health system unfolds, including the following:

  1. *Teacher training.* High-quality staff development, a key factor in effective education, is especially needed for health education. The teacher must have a good understanding of the content, a sensitivity to and enthusiasm for nurturing the health of each student, and an ability and willingness to model healthy living. New teachers, including all elementary teachers, must be adequately prepared to teach this area of the curriculum by taking an accredited university course dealing with teaching health education. High school teachers who teach a specific health class or who teach health as part of a home economics or science course also need special preservice preparation and training.

     In addition, all those teaching health need continuing professional development opportunities so that they can maintain their knowledge of current health topics and successful instructional strategies. Each district should ensure that teachers have sufficient opportunities for professional development in health education.

  2. *Training for other staff.* Nonteaching staff at the school, such as secretaries, school maintenance personnel, and classroom assistants, interact with and influence young people. The entire staff should be offered training in the philosophy of the coordinated school health system and their roles in helping students develop lifelong healthy behaviors. In addition, opportunities for cross-training with school-linked health and human-services providers will greatly strengthen the coordinated school health system. Training of this type is consistent with and may be a part of efforts to restructure schools. The major California school reform documents challenge schools to look at the entire curriculum and the environment of the school to ensure that all students succeed. Involvement of staff members in the coordinated school health system supports that goal.

  3. *Training and informational presentations for parents.* Parents should be offered opportunities to learn more about the content of the health education curriculum and the philosophy behind the coordinated school health system. They should understand the range of topics in the curriculum and should also have access to content.

- *Keep the vision in focus.* Once there is commitment to the vision and broad-based input, planning for further implementation of the components of a coordinated school health system should be a continuing process. Developing, evaluating, and refining specific goals and objectives for the coordinated school health system will ensure that the vision remains at the heart of the effort. Many schools will have some components of a coordinated school health system already in place and functioning well, others will be in place but in need of change, and still others will not yet be under way. Strategic thinking and planning will be needed, but the vision of a comprehensive approach will be the essential guide.

A quality health education curriculum supported by the components of a coordinated school health system with high visibility, effective monitoring, and qualified and enthusiastic participants is not an impossible goal. Although planning and implementation will take time and thoughtful effort, a coordinated school health system can be achieved when families, communities, and schools work together and make the health of children and youths a priority.

Chapter 2
Developing Health
Literacy in the
Classroom and
in the School

Meeting these challenges is the only wise course toward securing the future of the nation. But more than that, it is the right and moral thing to do for our young people, and we must accept nothing less.

—Code Blue: Uniting for
Healthier Youth

School Policies on Health Issues

A clearly stated policy that defines the coordinated school health system and expresses support for this system can greatly facilitate effective implementation. Specific district policies on a variety of health-related issues can be reviewed for their consistency with the coordinated school health system and incorporated into this policy. Addressing all health issues in one board policy helps ensure consistency and facilitates review and revision when necessary.

Districts developing policies for the first time or districts updating policies may wish to consider the California State Board of Education's policy on nutrition and state law regarding tobacco-free policies. These policies are summarized below:

Policy on Nutrition

The State Board of Education recommends that local educational agency and county office governing boards adopt policies that address all of the following issues:

1. A statement summarizing the district's or county office's nutrition policy
2. A plan for policy implementation and enforcement
3. A description of the local enforcement procedure

The policy should apply to all school-approved groups, including but not limited to students, teachers, parents, booster groups, and outside vendors. It would be appropriate for elementary school policies to be more restrictive than those for junior and senior high schools. Local policies that are more restrictive than existing state or federal laws and regulations are also acceptable.

Tobacco-Free Policies

"All school districts and county offices of education . . . shall adopt smoke-free campus policies and shall prohibit the use of tobacco on

(Continued on next page)

Chapter 2
Developing Health
Literacy in the
Classroom and
in the School

school property no later than July 1, 1996" (*Health and Safety Code* Section 24167[q][2]). A fully implemented tobacco-free policy includes the following:

- Policy prohibits the use of tobacco products anywhere, anytime on county or district property and in county or district vehicles.
- Enforcement procedures are established.
- Information about the policy and enforcement procedures are communicated clearly to county, district, or school personnel, parents, students, and the larger community.
- Signs stating the prohibition of tobacco use are prominently displayed at all entrances to county, district, or school property.
- A referral program to smoking cessation support programs is made available, and students and staff are encouraged to participate.

Chapter 2
Developing Health
Literacy in the
Classroom and
in the School

Importance of Research-Based Programs

Elementary and secondary education in recent years have seen an increasing emphasis placed on higher standards, accountability, and results. Given this new educational environment, effective, research-based programs and curricula have become as important to school health programs as they are to any other curricular area.

Several health education topics, including tobacco, alcohol and other drugs, nutrition, and human immunodeficiency virus/acquired immunodeficiency syndrome (HIV/AIDS), have received categorical funding. The requirements of such funding, of course, include accountability for program effectiveness. The Centers for Disease Control and Prevention (CDC), through its Division of Adolescent and School Health (DASH), has a particular interest in prevention programs that address risk factors known to be the major causes of morbidity and mortality in the United States. From 1992 to 2002 DASH undertook a process to identify effective prevention programs for youths. The process focused on the prevention of HIV/AIDS, sexually transmitted diseases (STDs), pregnancy, and tobacco use. Curricula that provided credible evidence of effectiveness were called "Programs That Work."

The following criteria were among those required for inclusion in Programs That Work:

- The intervention was a complete curricular program or package, not just a single component, such as a video.
- The intervention involved a classroom or other group setting.
- Content areas were specific to the program's health focus (e.g., tobacco-use prevention or STD prevention).
- The study population was composed of school-age youths (particularly middle school through high school for HIV, STD, and pregnancy prevention curricula).
- The research design included an intervention group and a control or comparison group.
- Follow-up measurement took place at least four weeks after the HIV, STD, or pregnancy prevention intervention ended or at least six months after the tobacco-use intervention ended.
- A report of the study had been published or accepted for publication in a peer-reviewed journal (e.g., a professional publication focusing on school health, psychology, or drug-abuse prevention).
- The study measured specific risk behaviors and health outcomes related to the content areas.
- The results found an association between exposure to the intervention and at least one specifically defined positive outcome related to the targeted health-risk behavior.
- The curriculum could be used by the average teacher, with appropriate training.

Chapter 2
Developing Health
Literacy in the
Classroom and
in the School

During the Programs That Work review process, CDC appointed a panel of evaluation experts to assess the validity of the program's evaluation and a panel of program experts to assess the feasibility of replicating the program. If both panels recommended adoption, CDC designated the curriculum as a Program That Works.

In California a similar Department of Education initiative has been the development of a series of guides and professional literature reviews under the general rubric of *Getting Results* (see Additional References and Resources). Established in conjunction with the federally funded Safe and Drug-Free Schools and Communities program and the state-funded Tobacco-Use Prevention Education program, *Getting Results* emphasizes the need for careful selection of research-based practices. The following criteria are among those that can be used for the selection of an effective, research-based health curriculum or program:

- The program is based on a theory that is accepted by experts.
- The theory provides a logical explanation of why the program should work.
- The program has produced the desired changes in the target population.
- The research has been conducted by reputable researchers and published in a reputable journal (preferably a peer-reviewed journal).
- The study has used a rigorous evaluation design.
- The study shows few negative effects.
- The study has been replicated at more than one site.
- The program has been implemented by school staff in the study.
- The students in the study are similar to students in the district selecting the curriculum or program.
- The program appears to be cost-effective.

Districts and schools are well advised to ensure that health instruction is based on current and confirmed research and complies with *Education Code* mandates. Therefore, the process of selecting and implementing programs that fit the criteria noted above requires great care. Establishing a good match between what a particular program offers and the school district's unique needs is a central element of that process. "No single curriculum or scientifically validated prevention strategy," writes education researcher J. Fred Springer, "will replace the skill and judgment of program designers and deliverers in constructing programs that make sense in their schools and communities."[2]

---

[2] J. Fred Springer, "Beyond the Magic Bullet: How We Can Achieve Science-Based Prevention," in *Getting Results, Update 1: Positive Youth Development: Research, Commentary, and Action.* Sacramento: California Department of Education, 1999, p. 39.

43

Chapter 2
Developing Health
Literacy in the
Classroom and
in the School

Life Skills and Positive Behaviors

Traditional health education has relied heavily on providing students with relevant health knowledge. The assumption has been that unhealthy behavior is the result of ignorance, but research does not support this assumption.[3] For example, a meta-analysis of smoking prevention programs for adolescents showed that the effects of traditional or "rational" approaches to influencing health behavior were small and insignificant.[4]

Recent research on HIV/AIDS, smoking, and drug use has shown that the inclusion of personal and social skills development is an effective approach for attaining positive health behavior.[5] Further credibility for emphasizing personal and social skills development can be found in a social influences model.[6] This model recognizes and emphasizes the social environment as a critical factor in shaping health behavior. Influences such as the family, school, the faith community, cultural contexts, peer behavior, and media are of great importance.

The implications of this research are that health education should not only provide relevant health knowledge but also build the skills students need to recognize and resist negative influences. These skills need to be both personal (intrapersonal) and social (interpersonal). Skills development should include but not be limited to analysis of media messages, decision making, coping strategies, assertiveness, refusal skills, validation of perceived social norms, and resolution of conflicts. To a great extent, the development of personal and social skills has been missing from health education. That shortcoming has resulted in ineffective efforts to promote positive health behavior.

---

[3] B. R. Flay, "Psychosocial Approaches to Smoking Prevention: A Review of Findings," *Health Psychology,* Vol. 4, No. 5 (1985), 449–88; P. M. Lantz and others, "Investing in Youth Tobacco Control: A Review of Smoking Prevention and Control Strategies," *Tobacco Control,* Vol. 9 (2000), 47–63.

[4] W. H. Bruvold, "A Meta-Analysis of Adolescent Smoking Prevention Programs," *American Journal of Public Health,* Vol. 83 (1993), 872–80.

[5] T. Baranowski, C. L. Perry, and G. S. Parcel, "How Individual Environments and Health Behavior Interact: Social Cognitive Theory," in *Health Behavior and Health Education.* Edited by K. Glanz, F. M. Lewis, and B. K. Rimer. San Francisco: Jossey-Bass, Inc., 1997; S. I. Donaldson and others, "Resistance Skill Training and Onset of Alcohol Use: Evidence for Beneficial and Potentially Harmful Effects in Public and in Private Catholic Schools," *Health Psychology,* Vol. 14 (1995), 291–300; W. B. Hansen and R. B. McNeal, "Drug Education Practice: Results of an Observational Study," *Health Education Research: Theory and Practice,* Vol. 14, No. 1 (1999), 85–97; N. S. Tobler and H. H. Stratton, "Effectiveness of School-Based Drug Prevention Programs: A Meta-Analysis of the Research," *Journal of Primary Prevention,* Vol. 18, No. 1 (1997), 71–128.

[6] A. Bandura, *Social Foundations of Thought and Action.* Englewood Cliffs, N.J.: Prentice Hall, 1986; G. C. Homans, *Elementary Forms of Social Behavior* (Second edition). New York: Harcourt Brace Jovanovich, 1974; W. McGuire, "Social Psychology," in *New Horizons in Psychology.* Edited by P. C. Dodwell. Middlesex, England: Penguin Books, 1972; S. Schinke, B. Blythe, and L. Gilchrest, "Cognitive-Behavioral Prevention of Adolescent Pregnancy," *Journal of Counseling Psychology,* Vol. 28 (1981), 451–54; Mark K. Smith, *Paulo Freire.* The Home of Informal Education Web site. *<http://www.infed.org/thinkers/et-freir.htm>.* 1997.

Chapter 2
Developing Health
Literacy in the
Classroom and
in the School

Researchers William B. Hansen and Ralph B. McNeal offer the following insights on the state-of-the-art research on substance abuse, delinquency, and other high-risk behaviors.[7] A key feature of the research is its focus on the characteristics known broadly as risk and protective factors. Health education in California is at a stage of development in which considerable effort and expertise are required of educators to make programs work as they are intended to work. To create programs using life skills or social influence, researchers spend their time investigating which risk factors and protective factors are important targets for change and how those changes should be accomplished. Not all risk or protective factors are equal. New studies reinforce the concept that prevention is often the result of changing only a limited number of factors. Some examples of promising factors include peer norms, a sense of bonding to school, a commitment to avoid risk behaviors, and tolerance toward others. Programs that target these factors hold great promise for effective prevention of risk behaviors.

Health Education Planning and Development

School health programs and systems vary widely from one school district to another and may also differ among individual schools within a district. Perhaps the most important aspect of any school health program is the leadership, which depends on persons who are convinced of the importance of school health to academic achievement and are willing to be champions for effective program planning and implementation.

A variety of resources for planning and developing school health programs are widely available throughout California. The use of these resources in conjunction with the *Health Framework* and *Education Code* requirements will help schools establish a unified and coherent school health program.

Resources for Program Planning

In addition to the resources identified in other sections of this framework, many locally available resources may be considered in planning the program. These include the following:

- **Community resources**—local health departments, law enforcement agencies, state agencies, services for children and families, libraries, community health information centers, and county offices of education
- **School district resources**—school board members who are advocates of student health and well-being; nutrition specialists; and district staff responsible for curriculum, instruction, and staff development

---

[7] W. B. Hansen and R. B. McNeal, "Drug Education Practice: Results of an Observational Study," *Health Education Research: Theory and Practice,* Vol. 14, No. 1 (1999), 85–97.

45

Chapter 2
Developing Health
Literacy in the
Classroom and
in the School

- **School site resources**—administrators, teachers, librarians, and school psychologists who are personally involved in and committed to health and well-being; health teachers; physical education teachers; school nurses; and representatives of special-interest school organizations, such as Future Nurses and Friday Night Live
- **Family resources**—family members working in the health professions; family members who coach local sports teams; and families whose children have special health needs

The Health Curriculum

Intended as an aid to curriculum planning, the information in Chapter 3 of this framework presents the scope and sequence of health instruction together with grade-span descriptions and grade-level emphases. Other aids to curriculum planning are as follows:

- *Education Code.* The *Education Code* (*EC*) contains legislated requirements related to health education that should be incorporated into the curriculum planning process (see Appendix A).

- State-adopted instructional materials. The State Board of Education approves new or revised curricular materials for health education on a regular basis, usually once every seven years. All materials adopted by the State Board since 1995 are available for loan and review at no charge from the Healthy Kids Resource Center, 313 W. Winton Avenue, Room 180, Hayward, CA 94544-1187; (510) 670-4583; *<http:// www.californiahealthykids.org>*.

- School library resources and support. The public school library continues to evolve into an active and technology-rich environment sustained by the power of information. Information literacy is knowing how to access and use that information and is the foundation of lifelong learning. The school library provides a wealth of resources, both print and online, that support the health curriculum. In addition, professional school library media teachers are trained to conduct collaborative information literacy instruction. The process of analyzing, applying, evaluating, and interpreting health-related information, products, and services is an important part of information literacy training.

  Examples of these skills and behaviors that build sequentially are highlighted in Chapter 3 and include a variety of critical-thinking skills for reading and interpreting information as well as skills for analyzing and applying criteria to various ideas. The school library can provide a wealth of resources and strategies.[8]

---

[8] *Information Power: Building Partnerships for Learning.* Chicago: American Library Association, 1998.

Chapter 2
Developing Health
Literacy in the
Classroom and
in the School

Health Literacy Assessment

Assessment is an integral component of a health education program. Chapter 5 of this framework provides guidelines for the assessment of health literacy and states, "A wide array of assessment methods and instruments that measure behavior and skill development and support critical thinking and a student-centered curriculum should be used to assess student health literacy" (p. 217). Under the leadership of national organizations, such as the Centers for Disease Control and Prevention (CDC) and the Council of Chief State School Officers (CCSSO), several important health education standards and assessment initiatives have emerged. One such initiative is the CCSSO State Collaborative on Assessment of Student Standards (SCASS). This collaborative includes health education experts from throughout the country.

The CCSSO-SCASS Health Education Assessment Project's *Assessing Health Literacy: Assessment Framework* provides invaluable information for building a foundation to support a quality comprehensive health education program.[9] The document provides the overall infrastructure for developing all assessment items. It prioritizes skills and concepts for health education *assessment,* not instruction. California's *Health Framework* closely parallels the National Health Education Standards. The national standards, along with CDC's six priority adolescent risk behaviors, provided the driving forces for the development of *Assessing Health Literacy.* Table 1, "Relationship Between Health Education and Adolescent Risk Behaviors," illustrates the relationship between the *Health Framework*'s recommended health education content areas, the four unifying ideas and related student expectations, and the priority risk behaviors identified by CDC.

Cost, personnel, and time constraints make it impossible to assess all of the content delivered within a given health education curriculum. *Assessing Health Literacy* organizes assessment items at the elementary, middle, and high school levels for skills and concepts that are most likely to yield health-promoting behaviors among youths. A total of more than 2,800 items have been developed and tested. The types of items used in the project include selected response (multiple choice), constructed response (short answer/extended response), performance events, and performance tasks.

---

[9] *Assessing Health Literacy: Assessment Framework.* Prepared by the Council of Chief State School Officers. Soquel, Calif.: ToucanEd Publications, 1998.

Table 1
Relationship Between Health Education and Adolescent Risk Behaviors

Health Education Content Areas	Unifying Ideas and Student Expectations Promoted in the *Health Framework*	Adolescent Risk Behaviors Identified by Centers for Disease Control and Prevention
Personal health	*Unifying Idea: Acceptance of Personal Responsibility for Lifelong Health*	Behaviors that result in intentional and unintentional injury
Consumer and community health	1. Students will demonstrate ways in which they can enhance and maintain their health and well-being.	Use of alcohol and other drugs
Injury prevention and safety	2. Students will demonstrate behaviors that prevent disease and speed recovery from illness.	Sexual behaviors that result in HIV infection, other STDs, or unintended pregnancy
Alcohol, tobacco, and other drugs	3. Students will practice behaviors that reduce the risk of becoming involved in potentially dangerous situations and react to potentially dangerous situations in ways that help to protect their health.	Tobacco use
Nutrition	*Unifying Idea: Respect for and Promotion of the Health of Others*	Dietary patterns that contribute to disease
Environmental health	1. Students will play a positive, active role in promoting the health of their families.	Sedentary lifestyle
Family living	2. Students will promote positive health practices within the school and community, including developing positive relationships with their peers.	
Individual growth and development	*Unifying Idea: An Understanding of the Process of Growth and Development*	
Communicable and chronic diseases	1. Students will understand the variety of physical, mental, emotional, and social changes that occur throughout life.	
	2. Students will understand and accept individual differences in growth and development.	
	3. Students will understand their developing sexuality, will choose to abstain from sexual activity, will learn about protecting their sexual health, and will treat the sexuality of others with respect.	
	Unifying Idea: Informed Use of Health-Related Information, Products, and Services	
	Students will identify information, products, and services that may be helpful or harmful to their health.	

Chapter 2
Developing Health
Literacy in the
Classroom and
in the School

Implications for Health Literacy Assessment

The information provided in *Assessing Health Literacy* can help educators direct health literacy education accountability systems in the following ways:

- Conduct needs assessments for health instruction.
- Establish baseline data regarding student health literacy.
- Measure the extent to which the *Health Framework*'s grade-level expectations have been achieved.
- Align the *Health Framework,* classroom instruction, and assessment methodologies.
- Facilitate the transition from teaching health knowledge to teaching health skills.
- Develop an assessment system that reflects improvements in students' health-related knowledge and skills.
- Evaluate the effectiveness of programs.

CCSSO has developed a series of CD-ROMs that present all the assessment items, examples, rubrics, and skill cards discussed in *Assessing Health Literacy.* The CD-ROMs and other related resources are available for loan from the Healthy Kids Resource Center.

Involvement of Other Health Experts

When planning a health education curriculum, leaders should keep in mind that many professionals with special health-related expertise and interest are available in schools and communities. Potential human resources include health care providers; public health educators in tobacco, alcohol, and drug prevention; public health nurses; juvenile justice staff; environmental health specialists; mental health counselors; and nutritionists.

Opportunities for student involvement in health issues in the community can be added to the curriculum through these experts' participation in the learning experience. When guests are invited to participate in the classroom, school policies should be considered and adequate precautions taken to ensure student safety and the guests' adherence to curriculum standards and practices.

Needs of Special Populations

The mission of the California Department of Education is to provide leadership, assistance, oversight, and resources so that every Californian has access to an education that meets world-class standards. Some students face barriers that impede learning or access to educational, health-related resources. Educators and administrators must make accommodations to minimize the impact of those barriers on students' education. The most commonly affected populations are students with exceptional needs, expectant and parenting teens,

49

Chapter 2
Developing Health
Literacy in the
Classroom and
in the School

homeless children and youths, and foster children and youths. Guidelines to accommodate those students are as follows:

Education for Students with Exceptional Needs

The United States Congress has declared that "Disability is a natural part of the human experience and in no way diminishes the right of individuals to participate in or contribute to society. Improving educational results for children with disabilities is an essential element of our national policy of ensuring equality of opportunity, full participation, independent living, and economic self-sufficiency for individuals with disabilities" (Individuals with Disabilities Education Act, 1997, Part A, Section 601[c][1]).

Advances in science and technology, in conjunction with society's increased commitment to promoting optimal learning and development for all children, have increased opportunities for students with exceptional needs to better realize their own potential. However, these advances bring with them substantial challenges for families, schools, communities, and society as a whole. To meet the challenges in an effective, efficient, and safe manner, experts in education, health, social services, law, financing, and municipal services must collaborate with families and communities to identify and promote practices and programs that will enhance the quality of life for these students.

The protection of education rights for students with exceptional needs is guaranteed by the following legislation:

- Public Law 94-142, passed in 1975, renamed the Individuals with Disabilities Education Act (IDEA) in 1990, and reauthorized in 1997 (20 *United States Code [USC]* sections 1400 et seq.; and 34 *Code of Federal Regulations [CFR]*, parts 300 and 303)
- The federal Rehabilitation Act, Section 504 (29 *USC* 705 [20] and 794; and 34 *CFR*, Part 104)
- The federal Americans with Disabilities Act (ADA) (42 *USC* 12101– 12213; 47 *USC* 225 and 611; and 28 *CFR*, Part 35)
- *Education Code*, Part 30 (Section 56000 et seq.)
- *California Code of Regulations, Title 5* (Section 3000 et seq.)
- *Government Code*, Chapter 26.5 (Section 7570 et seq.)

Of the three federal legislative pieces, only IDEA is specific to education. Section 504 of the Rehabilitation Act and ADA are civil rights legislation concerned with discrimination and equal access and, as such, guarantee students with disabilities an education comparable to that provided to nondisabled students.

Note: Staff development programs must be provided for regular and special education teachers, administrators, certificated and classified employees, volunteers, community advisory committee members, and, as appropriate,

Chapter 2
Developing Health
Literacy in the
Classroom and
in the School

members of the district and county governing boards. Such programs shall include, but not be limited to, the provision of opportunities for all school personnel, paraprofessionals, and volunteers to participate in ongoing development activities pursuant to a systematic identification of pupil and personnel needs *(Education Code* sections 56240 and 56241[a]).

Other resources related to special education programs are as follows:

- "California Special Education Programs: A Composite of Laws Database," *Education Code,* Part 30, Other Related Laws, and *California Code of Regulations, Title 5* at *<http://www.cde.ca.gov/spbranch/sed/ lawsreg2.htm>*
- *A Composite of Laws, California Special Education Programs, 25th Edition* (Sacramento: California Department of Education, 2003)
- The California Law Web site at *<http://www.leginfo.ca.gov/calaw.html>*
- *California Code of Regulations* Web site at *<http://ccr.oal.ca.gov>*
- *United States Code* Web site at *<http://uscode.house.gov/usc.htm>*
- *Code of Federal Regulations* Web site at *<http://www.access.gpo.gov/ nara/cfr/ >*

Expectant and Parenting Teens

Teen pregnancy is one of the most pressing and poignant problems facing society and carries personal and social costs. It is a complex issue of physical, social, cultural, and economic factors that hold myriad ramifications for individuals, families, communities, the state, and the nation.

According to the State Superintendent of Public Instruction's *Report to the Legislature,* teen pregnancy presents challenges not only to teens, their children, and their families, but also to state and local governments and society as a whole in terms of strained resources.[10] Many challenges facing the educational system are caused by the following conditions:

- Pregnancy and parenting responsibilities are the number-one reason that females drop out of school.
- A high correlation exists between low basic skills and teen pregnancy.
- A high correlation exists between low birth weight in infants and the need for special education services.
- Pregnancy among females younger than fifteen years of age is increasing.

The California School Age Families Education (Cal-SAFE) Program, established by Chapter 1078, Statutes of 1998, became operational in July 2000. This comprehensive, community-linked, school-based program is designed to increase the availability of support services necessary for enrolled expectant and parenting students to improve their academic achievement and parenting skills and to provide a quality child care and development program

[10] Delaine Eastin, *A Report to the Legislature.* Sacramento: California Department of Education, 1996.

51

Chapter 2
Developing Health
Literacy in the
Classroom and
in the School

for their children. Cal-SAFE builds on education reform initiatives, ensures a quality education program with high standards for enrolled students, and mandates accountability of local educational agencies for the performance of students and their children in meeting program goals. Comprehensive health education is one of the allowable expenditures of Cal-SAFE Program funds. More information is available on CDE's Cal-SAFE Program Web site at <*http://www.cde.ca.gov/calsafe*>.

Through existing school resources or collaboration with community partners, such as the Adolescent Family Life Program (AFLP) and the Cal-Learn Program, schools can coordinate strategies to help expectant and parenting students gain access to such necessary support services as perinatal care, child care, and transportation between home and school. Strategies for addressing these students' special needs are as follows:

- *Health education.* Pregnancy and subsequent parenthood call attention to the need for health education for teen parents and health care for their children and for themselves. In addition to being more aware of their own bodies' needs, pregnant teens and also teen mothers and fathers should be concerned and have knowledge about the health of their children. An effective strategy to meet this need is to modify the content areas of the health education curriculum to focus on the priorities and unique needs of expectant and parenting students. For example, tobacco prevention education is more relevant when discussed in terms of the effects of smoking on teens' unborn children and the effects of secondhand smoke on children. Expectant and parenting teens are facing adult responsibilities, and this period in their lives holds an opportunity for them to develop lifelong healthy habits and act as positive role models for their children.

- *Nutritious meal supplements, education, and counseling.* Good nutrition is a crucial part of prenatal and postnatal care. Pregnancy intensifies the nutritional needs of teenagers, increasing in particular the need for calcium, protein, and certain vitamins and minerals. Poor diet and improper weight gain or loss on the part of pregnant teens can lead to poor outcomes, such as premature and low-birth-weight babies. Teen mothers must make sound nutrition decisions for the well-being of their children. Teen parents also need to know about appropriate feeding patterns, including breastfeeding, for their children as they move through the infant, toddler, and preschool stages. Teen parents must develop responsible, healthful eating habits in order to provide good role models for their children.

- *Physical education program.* One of the most neglected aspects of a pregnant or parenting student's educational experience is the teen's physical education/fitness program. With physician approval, pregnant

Chapter 2
Developing Health
Literacy in the
Classroom and
in the School

women can engage in a moderate level of physical activity to maintain cardiorespiratory and muscular fitness throughout pregnancy and the postpartum period. An individualized physical education/fitness program should be developed for each teen under the direction of a physician to promote the pregnant teen's safe engagement in physical activity that strengthens and tones muscles, increases stamina and endurance, and improves general health.

The major considerations in the design of a modified physical education/ fitness program related to pregnancy include (1) regulation of body temperature (remain well hydrated and avoid exercise in high heat or humidity); (2) avoidance of a supine position in the mid and late stages of pregnancy (perform abdominal exercises while standing or on hands and knees); (3) limitation of the range of motion (avoid heavy lifting and high-impact activities); and (4) recognition of the change in center of gravity, which may cause balance problems and the risk of falling (avoid activities requiring sudden changes in direction or position).

- *Counseling/case management.* Teen pregnancy and teen parenting affect not only the teen parents and their children but also the adult parents of the teens, any siblings, and the extended family. This period is a time of profound change and may cause friction between the teen mother and the father of her child as well as between the families of the young parents. Schools may need to provide individual or family counseling either directly or through referral to a public or private mental health agency. Peer support groups and counseling may be available through school programs targeting the special needs of expectant and parenting students and their children. Support services for grandparents, siblings, and teen or adult fathers of babies born to teen mothers may be needed to promote success in school for the students.

- *Prenatal education and service referral.* Pregnant women, regardless of age, need early referral to prenatal education and care in order to promote positive birth outcomes for them and their children. Pregnant teens may delay seeking health care for a variety of reasons. School nurses and staff working in programs for pregnant and parenting students can promote positive birth outcomes by providing appropriate health education instruction, including reproductive health care, and by referring students to community agencies and programs that address the needs of pregnant women.

Children and Youths Living in Homeless Situations

In California an estimated 222,000 children and youths from birth to eighteen years of age live in homeless situations, as defined by *Education Code* Section 1981.2, during all or part of the school year. Students in this group

Chapter 2
Developing Health
Literacy in the
Classroom and
in the School

present special challenges to teachers, administrators, counselors, and other school staff. *Education Code* Section 48200, the compulsory attendance law, requires school attendance for children six to eighteen years of age. Federal law (No Child Left Behind [NCLB] Act of 2001 [PL103-382], Title I, Part A) requires local educational agencies to reserve funds to provide services, including education-related support services, to homeless children and youths who are eligible under Title I. The Stewart B. McKinney Homeless Assistance Act (PL 100-77) provides assistance to ensure that homeless youths have equal access to a free, appropriate public education. District policies and procedures must be in place to ensure that homeless children and youths are not denied the opportunity to enroll in, attend, and succeed in school.

Outreach and awareness are key components in overcoming barriers facing the education of homeless children and youths. School districts may assist with transportation services to encourage consistent attendance and instructional continuity. In-service training should be provided to district and school personnel to foster an understanding of the issues and needs facing homeless students and to create a positive learning environment for them. To enroll a child in school, families must meet certain requirements and provide appropriate documentation, conditions that often present obstacles for those living in homeless situations. School personnel may satisfy the enrollment requirements with alternative documents to facilitate the enrollment of homeless children and youths. Some of the conditions that must be met include residency requirements, placement in the school of origin or attendance, and the verification of documents. Records are required to verify birth date, grade level, up-to-date immunizations, parent or guardian, and emergency contacts. To verify that a child has received the necessary immunizations to enroll in school, schools need an immunization record from a health clinic, doctor, school, or social service agency. If the information is unobtainable, school officials should direct the family to the nearest health clinic or health provider. The parent or guardian should provide a medical release for the student and emergency notification information on the standard school emergency card. If a parent or guardian cannot be reached in an emergency, schools should follow normal policies and procedures in providing care for the student.

More information on issues affecting the education of children and youths living in homeless situations can be found in the publications *Enrolling Students Living in Homeless Situations* and *Pieces of the Puzzle: Creating Success for Students in Homeless Situations.*[11]

---

[11] *Enrolling Students Living in Homeless Situations.* Sacramento: California Department of Education, 1999; B. James and others, *Pieces of the Puzzle: Creating Success for Students in Homeless Situations.* Austin: University of Texas, 1997.

Chapter 2
Developing Health
Literacy in the
Classroom and
in the School

Foster Children and Youths

Foster Youth Services (FYS) programs provide support services to displaced students to reduce the traumatic effects of being removed from their families and schools and placed in unfamiliar home settings. The programs have the authority to ensure that health and school records are obtained to establish appropriate placements and coordinate instruction, counseling, tutoring, mentoring, vocational training, and emancipation services for foster children and youths. These services are designed to improve the children's educational performance and personal achievement.

Currently, approximately 105,000 to 110,000 children in California are in foster care. When foster children experience changes in care and school placement, they face the stresses of falling behind academically, losing academic credit, and losing contact with persons who are aware of their health and welfare needs. In 1999–2000 FYS projects served approximately 3,400 foster youths, and countywide programs provided services for approximately 13,000 foster youths residing in group homes. Data collected from providers of FYS programs demonstrate that these services have resulted in major quantitative improvements in pupil academic achievement, the incidence of pupil discipline problems or juvenile delinquency, and pupil dropout and truancy rates.

Schools are clearly a focal point for identifying foster children's academic and behavioral problems and needs. Through interagency collaboration providers of foster youth services work with social workers, probation officers, group home staff, school staff, and community service agencies to influence the day-to-day routines of foster children both during and after school. The Health and Education Passport (*Education Code* Section 49069.5) includes complete health and school records and is a tool for establishing appropriate placements and coordinating instruction, counseling, tutoring, mentoring, and other training and related services for foster youths. Accurate student information facilitates appropriate placement, increases the stability of placements, and ensures that children receive appropriate support services that improve their educational performance and personal achievement.

Additional information and resources or a copy of the *Report to the Governor and Legislature on Foster Youth Services Programs* (*Education Code* Section 42923), dated February 15, 2000, are available from the Educational Options Office, California Department of Education, telephone (916) 322-5012; Web site *<http://www.cde.ca.gov/spbranch>*.

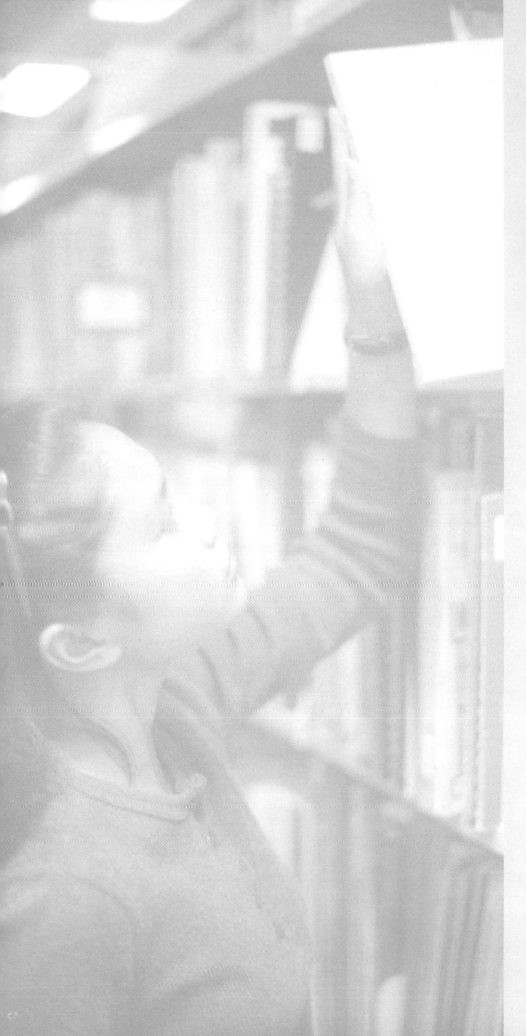

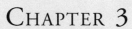
CHAPTER 3

Health
Education

I.
The Health Curriculum: An Overview

Health education is integral to a coordinated school health system. A well-designed health curriculum for students in kindergarten through grade twelve offers abundant opportunities for engaging students and involving them in meaningful learning experiences. The curriculum should provide students with opportunities to explore concepts in depth, analyze and solve real-life problems, and work cooperatively on tasks that develop and enhance their conceptual understanding. It also provides students with the knowledge and skills that can lead to lifelong positive attitudes and behaviors related to health.

The major goal of health education envisioned in this framework is the development of health literacy in all students. The four unifying ideas of health literacy emphasized throughout the health curriculum are the following:

- *Acceptance of personal responsibility,* including responsibility for personal lifelong health, acceptance of the idea that the individual has some control over health, and incorporation of health-related knowledge into everyday behavior
- *Respect for and promotion of the health of others,* including an understanding and acceptance of the influence of behavior on the health and well-being of others, of people on the environment, and of the environment on the health of groups and individuals
- *An understanding of the process of growth and development,* including the importance of both universal and individual aspects of physical, mental, emotional, and social growth and development
- *Informed use of health-related information, products, and services,* including the ability to select and use health-related information, products, and services carefully and wisely

A curriculum that addresses the four unifying ideas will draw content from the nine major content areas of health education:

- Personal Health
- Consumer and Community Health
- Injury Prevention and Safety
- Alcohol, Tobacco, and Other Drugs

- Nutrition
- Environmental Health
- Family Living
- Individual Growth and Development
- Communicable and Chronic Diseases

The content areas are the traditional, widely used subject categories of health education. With minor variations they have appeared consistently in previous California frameworks and in other state and national descriptions of comprehensive health education. Together, the content areas describe the range of health concepts, skills, and behaviors important for today's students. In the course of a year, most if not all of the content areas should be included in the curriculum. To be woven throughout the content areas are the concepts related to mental and emotional health. Basic to all parts of health education, those concepts are to be included in the curriculum each year.

The content areas are not distinct from the four unifying ideas of health literacy. Rather, the unifying ideas run through and connect the content areas in a student-centered approach that makes instruction meaningful to students. A well-designed health curriculum combines the four unifying ideas with the content areas in a continuing spiral of knowledge and skill development from kindergarten through grade twelve. This chapter presents the broad outlines of such a program.

II.
Content Areas, Kindergarten Through Grade Twelve

The following descriptions of the nine content areas apply across grade levels from kindergarten through grade twelve. Expectations and content for specific ranges of grade levels can be found in Section III.

Personal Health

Personal health lays the foundation for good general health. Instruction in personal health encourages a positive commitment to health and well-being rooted in respect for oneself and one's physical, mental, emotional, and social health. Understanding that exercise is essential to good health, a person realizes that to stay healthy and fit is basic to personal health.

Three ideas are central to personal health. First, good health is not simply a matter of luck or accident; it involves taking responsibility and making deliberate choices. Second, good health involves an interaction of physical, mental, emotional, and social aspects of health, reflecting the interdependence of body and mind. Third, a commitment to personal health is one basis for leading a happy, healthy, productive life.

Consumer and Community Health

As a nation we face a growing concern about the cost of health care and the need to focus on health promotion and disease prevention. Addressing that concern implies a shift not only in how health-care services are provided but also in how individuals take an active role in deciding on their use of health-care services and health-related products.

Three main ideas are central to this content area. First, the age-old principle of buyer beware is particularly relevant to health-related decisions. In many cases medical problems may get better without treatment or with simple treatment at home. When skilled health care is needed, one should know how to find the appropriate services and avoid products or services that may be useless or even harmful. Second, preventing illness and promoting health are in the best interest of both individuals and society. Third, a variety of community organizations and agencies are available to assist those experiencing problems.

Injury Prevention and Safety

However childhood injury is measured (in number of deaths, dollar costs for treatment, relative rankings with other health problems, or loss of potential years of life), it ranks first among health problems affecting children in California and the nation. Historically, although childhood mortality due to disease has been reduced dramatically, that due to injury has increased steadily. Unintentional injuries, mainly those involving motor vehicles but also those caused by drowning, fire, suffocation, or poisoning, together with intentional injuries resulting from violent behavior, rank among the greatest threats to the health of children and young adults.

Yet the causes of injuries can be prevented or avoided. This content area focuses on prevention through safe living habits and positive, healthy decisions. Simple precautions and an awareness of the consequences of one's choices and decisions can help to prevent many unintentional injuries. This content area also acknowledges that violence is a public health issue. The curriculum at all grade levels should include a comprehensive approach to the prevention of violence.

Another focus of this content area is knowing what to do when confronted with emergencies. Appropriate responses are critically important in emergencies resulting from natural disasters or the actions of dangerous persons.

Note: See summary of *Education Code* Section 51202 (personal and public health and safety) in Appendix A. The requirements of this code section should be understood prior to the development of curriculum in this content area.

Violence is a public health issue. The curriculum at all grade levels should include a comprehensive approach to the prevention of violence.

Alcohol, Tobacco, and Other Drugs

The use of alcohol, tobacco, and other drugs, so pervasive and so potentially damaging to the health of individuals and society, has major implications in the lifelong health of individuals. Successful efforts to prevent the use of tobacco are effective against four of the five leading causes of death in California: heart disease, cancer, chronic obstructive lung disease, and fire caused by smoking.

A multifaceted approach, including a full range of prevention and intervention components, is required to safeguard the health of students from the effects of alcohol, tobacco, and other drugs. As a starting point information should be presented on the effects of alcohol, tobacco, including smokeless tobacco and secondhand smoke, and other drugs on the body. Information should also be presented on all types of drugs, including medicines and such performance-enhancing substances as steroids. The proper use of medication and the role of medication in the treatment of disease are key concepts. The effects of alcohol, tobacco, and other drugs on pregnant women and their children should also be addressed, together with the social effects of their use and the relation of alcohol and drug use to suicide, violence, and other health and safety issues.

A multifaceted approach, including a full range of prevention and intervention components, is required to safeguard the health of students from the effects of alcohol, tobacco, and other drugs.

As important as the development of knowledge related to alcohol, tobacco, and other drugs is the need for young people to develop skills in resisting the influence of peers and the media to use legal and illegal substances that are potentially harmful. With so many health-related choices influenced by peers, skill-building activities, such as development of refusal and communication skills, are a necessary component of instruction at all grade levels. Students should know that the consumption of alcohol and the use of tobacco and other drugs (with the exception of appropriate medications) are prohibited at school and should be familiar with the consequences for failure to comply.

The environment in which alcohol, tobacco, and other drugs are made available must also be considered. Society accepts the adult use of tobacco and alcohol, sending conflicting messages to young people regarding their use. As a result children must be prepared to deal with situations in which they cannot control the use of alcohol, tobacco, and other drugs by others. To strengthen the school's message and provide for consistency at home and in the community, parents and other members of the community should be involved in developing curriculum and intervention strategies designed to prevent the use of alcohol, tobacco, and other drugs and should be encouraged to support the school's no-use message to students. They should work together to identify and reduce specific risks and increase protection.

Collaborative efforts are also helpful in refining and enhancing procedures for identification, assessment, referral, and ongoing support for children and youths who have previously used alcohol, tobacco, or other drugs and in providing information on available counseling, treatment, and reentry programs and services to students and employees. One important, appropriate function of community involvement is communicating information to parents and the community about problems with the use of alcohol, tobacco, and other drugs experienced by youths as well as effective strategies to prevent their use. In addition, community involvement brings law enforcement agencies and the community into the schools, builds bridges between the school and the community, and develops more effective communication and cooperative relationships. Through a well-coordinated effort, schools, families, law enforcement agencies, and the community can work together to develop, promote, and carry out a clear, unified position on the use of alcohol, tobacco, and other drugs.

Note: See summaries of *Education Code* sections 51202 (personal and public health and safety) and 51203 (alcohol, narcotics, restricted dangerous drugs, and other dangerous substances) in Appendix A. The requirements of these code sections should be understood prior to the development of curriculum in this content area.

Nutrition

To be ready to learn and to achieve their fullest potential, children need to be well nourished and healthy. For that reason they must have an adequate supply of healthy foods and the knowledge and skills required to make wise food choices. A primary issue for all children, then, especially the increasing number of children living in poverty, is access to an adequate diet. Effective nutrition education provides children and their families with information on gaining access to adequate food sources, including the range of school nutrition programs available.

Nutrition Services Specialists: Resources for Health Education

Often overlooked as health education or program resources are the professional nutritionists and registered dietitians affiliated with child nutrition programs. These nutrition specialists can provide tremendous resources. They and other child nutrition staff can help augment classroom activities and assist teachers with the integration of nutrition- or food-related activities with many subject areas and various schoolwide programs and services. Examples of such activities include:

- Providing assistance with mathematical calculations of the nutritional values of foods, recipes, and menus
- Developing consumer education skills, such as reading labels and getting the most for students' food dollars
- Increasing respect for other cultures and the foods of those cultures
- Providing assistance with lessons on the chemical reactions that take place in foods and lessons on safe food-handling practices and the relationship between food-handling and microbiology
- Providing assistance in developing disaster-preparedness plans and food kits for students
- Providing parent education in nutrition and food-related consumer practices
- Addressing the nutritional concerns of students with special health conditions

By including child nutrition professionals in programs and services, districts can maximize their resources and make the health team more comprehensive.

The link between nutrition and good health or, conversely, between poor nutrition and illness is another key concept. Healthy eating habits and an active lifestyle can increase resistance to communicable diseases and reduce the risk of chronic disease, developmental disabilities, and infant mortality, a particularly serious problem of teenage pregnancy. In California the basis for nutrition recommendations is the *California Daily Food Guide,*[1] which incorporates the federal dietary guidelines for Americans and the dietary recommendations of other national health authorities. Current nutrition recommendations are illustrated in the food guide pyramid developed by the U.S. Department of Agriculture.

Students learn that food choices are intimately linked with physical, mental, emotional, and social health; energy level; self-image; and physical fitness. This content area provides students with the knowledge, skills, and motivation needed to make wise food choices throughout their lives. Ideally, nutrition education uses the school's child nutrition programs as an essential part of the educational process. Food-tasting and preparation experiences at all grade levels can provide an excellent opportunity for classroom teachers to work cooperatively with school nutrition personnel and use the cafeteria as a learning laboratory for classroom lessons as required by federal and state legislation. (Public Law 95-166 provides funds to states for the development of comprehensive nutrition education programs that make full use of the school cafeteria.) One model nutrition curriculum is contained in the California Department of Education's *Choose Well, Be Well* series.[2]

Environmental Health

The primary focus of environmental health is to make students aware of how environmental issues affect their personal health. The content area also suggests specific steps that students can take as individuals and citizens to protect and improve the environment.

A number of health conditions are either caused or exacerbated by environmental factors. For example, asthma and other lung ailments can be aggravated by air pollutants; skin cancer, by unprotected exposure to the sun; intestinal disorders, by polluted water; and allergies, by pollens, dust, or animal dander. In addition, environmental teratogens, both naturally occurring and synthetic, can cause birth defects and developmental disabilities. Health hazards from air pollution, water pollution, excessive noise levels, unprotected sun exposure, and unhealthy working or living conditions are also unfortunate features of modern life.

---

[1] *The California Daily Food Guide.* Developed by the California Department of Health Services in collaboration with the California Department of Aging and the California Department of Education. Sacramento: California Department of Education, 1990.

[2] *Choose Well, Be Well* is a series of nutrition curriculum materials designed by teachers and nutrition experts for students in preschool through grade twelve, published 1982–84.

Students need to learn about health hazards resulting from the environment. They also need to be taught about the precautions and behaviors they can practice to safeguard their health from environmental hazards. This awareness should be combined with an awareness of practices that will reverse or at least slow down environmental pollution and related problems. Lessons that relate to recycling, conservation of resources, and an appreciation of the finite limits of environmental resources are important in this content area.

Note: See summary of *Education Code* Section 51202 (personal and public health and safety) in Appendix A. The requirement of this code section should be understood prior to the development of curriculum in this content area.

Family Living

In the teaching of family living, particular attention must be paid to the legislative codes and guidelines that affect curriculum planning and instruction within this content area. *Note:* See summaries of *Education Code* sections 51550 and 51555 (parent notification), 51553 (sex education course criteria, emphasizing abstinence), 51554 (parental notification of outside speakers for family life, AIDS, STDs), 51201.5 (HIV/AIDS prevention), and 51513 (personal beliefs) in Appendix A. The requirements of these code sections should be understood prior to the development of curriculum in this content area.

A functional family unit is vital to the well-being of children. Children usually develop best when they live in a stable environment with their mother and father and receive from their parents consistent love, support, and direction. However, children from nontraditional families can also develop successfully. Given the variety of nontraditional families in contemporary society, it is important that children not reared in two-parent families be convinced that their situation can also be conducive to growth and development.

Further, it is important that children not be denigrated because of their living arrangement or the composition of their family. All students, regardless of their current living arrangement, can benefit from classroom instruction and discussion on family living. They can learn how they can contribute to making the family unit harmonious and successful now as well as in the future—when they will likely become parents.

This content area promotes the development of positive family interactions in all types of families, including those that face unusual challenges. Families that have members with physical or mental disabilities can experience major effects on patterns of family interaction. Ideally, families can adapt to these challenges and in fact may develop stronger, more supportive family relationships as a result. Members of these families should feel comfortable participating in classroom discussions of family interactions.

Instruction in family living also focuses on sexuality, the reproductive process, dating relationships, and the selection of a mate. Abstinence from

Abstinence from sexual
activity is strongly
encouraged because it is
the healthiest course of
action for young people.

Because parents should
be the primary source of
sex education and values
relating to this subject,
they must be notified
before lessons in sex
education are offered.

sexual activity is strongly encouraged because it is the healthiest course of action for young people. Statistics based on the latest medical information citing the failure and success rates of condoms and other contraceptives in preventing pregnancy shall be provided to students. In addition, the moral, legal, and economic responsibilities of parenthood are highlighted.

Sexually transmitted diseases and their prevention are discussed. Because parents should be the primary source of sex education and values relating to this subject, they must be notified before lessons in sex education are offered. The *Education Code* permits parents to withdraw their children from this portion of the health curriculum.

Decisions regarding developing specific instruction in family living within the parameters of legal requirements rest with school districts. The approach of this framework is to encourage districts to work with parents and community members in developing curriculum, especially in the area of family living. The intent of the curriculum in this content area is not to invade the privacy of families and their right to teach values to their children but to assist families in teaching about family living and encourage effective family communication.

Because of the sensitive nature of this content area, school districts may wish to arrange same-sex groupings during presentation of this portion of the curriculum to younger students. Districts should work with parents and community members to decide how controversial issues such as homosexuality, abortion, and masturbation will, or will not, be addressed. Parents should be informed of the district's position, and teachers should receive clear training in fulfilling the district's policies.

Family life curricula must include factual, substantiated information that is free of racial, ethnic, and gender bias and, if consistent with district policy, an opportunity for students to explore different aspects of issues within the parameters allowed by law. The school district must determine what constitutes factual, substantiated information[3] and ensure that all instructional resources are subject to the district's review and approval process. If guest speakers are invited to participate in the discussion of those issues, the speakers' activities must be made to adhere to district policy and state law. Further, districts must ensure that schools comply with all legal requirements concerning family life education, including providing written notification to parents before conducting classes in which the human reproductive organs and their functions are described, illustrated, or discussed.[4]

---

[3] *Education Code* Section 51553(b): "(1)(A) Factual information presented in course material and instruction shall be medically accurate and objective. (B) For purposes of this section, the following definitions apply: (i) 'Factual information' includes, but is not limited to, medical, psychiatric, psychological, empirical, and statistical statements. (ii) 'Medically accurate' means verified or supported by research conducted in compliance with scientific methods and published in peer-review journals, where appropriate, and recognized as accurate and objective by professional organizations and agencies with expertise in the relevant fields such as the Centers for Disease Control and Prevention."

[4] School district governing boards dealing with policy issues should refer to Appendix A.

Individual Growth and Development

An important element of health is our view of ourselves and our sense of our relationship to those around us. This content area provides information about the wide range of patterns and rates of physical, mental, emotional, and social development that occur among children and young adults. This information includes the stages of the life cycle from conception through death, physical changes that occur during puberty, and changes in relationships with others that accompany social development and the aging process.

This content area encourages students to take pride in their personal identity. It teaches them to view self-esteem as being based not only on one's accomplishments but also on personal values and ethical considerations. Further, self-esteem frees one to make healthy decisions and refuse to take part in negative behaviors without the fear of rejection that may inhibit some individuals.

In addition, this content area focuses on the importance of positive interpersonal relationships as an element in individual health and well-being. Friendships are essential to a feeling of belonging and self-worth. Skills for sustaining long-term friendships can be cultivated, and friends can help each other make responsible decisions.

Finally, this content area addresses the growing number of physically or mentally challenged students being mainstreamed into regular classes and promotes their acceptance. As a result of mainstreaming, more children will be exposed to classmates with serious illness and may even experience the death of a classmate. Studying this content area will help students understand and respond appropriately to students with special needs.

Chances of contracting
most illnesses can be
greatly influenced by
students' health-related
choices and decisions. . . .
Sexually transmitted
diseases (STDs), including
HIV/AIDS and hepatitis B,
dramatically illustrate
this point.

Communicable and Chronic Diseases

The most important message to convey in this content area is that students have a considerable measure of control over their health and that chances of contracting most illnesses can be greatly influenced by students' health-related choices and decisions. Such communicable diseases as sexually transmitted diseases (STDs), including HIV/AIDS and hepatitis B, dramatically illustrate the point. Chances of contracting these diseases are greatly reduced when young people abstain from sexual activity and intravenous drug use and use universal precautions when dealing with other people's body fluids. *Note:* The importance of abstinence education is emphasized in the section on family living.

Although the effects of heredity must be considered, behaviors and decisions also affect the development of such chronic diseases as cardiovascular disease, cancer, hypertension and stroke, diabetes, and osteoporosis. The risk factors for these diseases can begin to be detected early in life and are greatly influenced by health-related choices. Communicable and chronic diseases are too often the consequences of short-sighted or uninformed choices.

With so many health-related choices influenced by peers, skill-building activities, such as development of refusal and communication skills, are a necessary component of instruction at all grade levels. Physically or mentally challenged children are especially susceptible to peer pressure and should be included in skill-building instruction and practice.

This content area also includes the skills necessary to act in a supportive yet safe manner toward people with diseases. Although it is important to promote tolerance toward people with disease, individuals and society also need to work to control and eradicate disease.

The discussion of sexually transmitted diseases and HIV infection and AIDS is a necessary and important part of this content area. *Note:* See summaries of *Education Code* sections 51550 (parent notification), 51553(a) (sex education course criteria, emphasizing abstinence), 51201.5 (HIV/AIDS prevention), and 51513 (personal beliefs) in Appendix A. The requirements of these code sections should be understood prior to the development of curriculum in this content area. As with the family life content area, parents must be notified before sex education classes are offered in which the human reproductive organs and their functions are described, illustrated, or discussed, including discussion of sexually transmitted diseases. Parents may withdraw their children from this portion of the health curriculum.

The discussion of communicable and chronic diseases can be sensitive and have cultural, socioeconomic, genetic, or religious implications. Although decisions regarding curriculum content rest with school districts, the approach of this framework is to encourage districts to work with parents and community members in developing the curriculum.

III.
Expectations and Content, by Grade Level

The four unifying ideas of health literacy and the related grade-span expectations are presented first. Then, in the new material, the grade-span expectations are organized into a chart indicating specific emphases for each elementary grade level and for middle school and high school.

Structure of the Instructional Guidelines for Each Grade

Each of the following sections introduces concepts and suggestions designed to facilitate the planning of curricula, instructional units, and instructional resources. Each section focuses on the four unifying ideas of health literacy and follows a specific format.

- Unifying idea: acceptance of personal responsibility for lifelong health; respect for and promotion of the health of others; an understanding of the process of growth and development; and informed use of health-related information, products, and services
- Grade-level expectations
- Concepts and content to be emphasized
- Examples of skills and behaviors to be taught and reinforced

Kindergarten Through Grade Three

Although much of their environment and daily living activities are beyond their control, students in kindergarten through grade three can choose many behaviors that contribute to good health. Because young children tend to be unself-consciously egocentric, a curriculum that focuses on them and on what they can do to promote their well-being captures their interest and attention. The curriculum should begin with the children and their immediate environment so that they can make clear connections to information, concepts, skills, and behaviors. It should also sustain a focus on the children's social development as members of the classroom, the school, families, and communities. Throughout, the prevention of unhealthy behaviors and promotion of attitudes and behaviors that can lead to lifelong health practices should be strongly emphasized.

Chapter 3
Health Education

III. Expectations
and Content,
by Grade Level

**Kindergarten
Through
Grade Three**

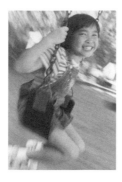

Unifying Idea

Acceptance of personal responsibility for lifelong health

Expectations:

1. Students will demonstrate ways in which they can enhance and maintain their health and well-being.
2. Students will understand and demonstrate behaviors that prevent disease and speed recovery from illness.
3. Students will practice behaviors that reduce the risk of becoming involved in potentially dangerous situations and react to potentially dangerous situations in ways that help to protect their health.

Expectation 1

Students will demonstrate ways in which they can enhance and maintain their health and well-being.

Grade-level concepts and content	*Examples of skills and behaviors*
The human body:	
Children at this level are curious about the function of body parts and their own bodies. Teaching them how their bodies function and the care required to maintain health empowers them to choose healthy behaviors. The curriculum should focus on habits related to physical care of the body and those related to protecting the body.	Practicing good personal hygiene, including caring for teeth, gums, eyes, ears, nose, skin, hair, and nails Using protective equipment or practicing behaviors to protect the body, such as: 1. Using a seat belt or helmet 2. Using sunscreen or a hat in bright sunlight 3. Keeping sharp objects away from one's eyes, ears, nose 4. Protecting ears from exposure to excessive noise 5. Wearing appropriate clothing and protective equipment for sports 6. Playing or exercising at times and in ways that minimize exposure to such environmental hazards as excessive heat and smog 7. Practicing ways to maintain correct posture and prevent back injuries

Chapter 3
Health Education

III. Expectations
and Content,
by Grade Level

**Kindergarten
Through
Grade Three**

Unifying Idea:
Acceptance of personal
responsibility for
lifelong health

Grade-level concepts and content	*Examples of skills and behaviors*

Food choices:

Because food preferences and dietary practices begin to be formed in childhood, students should begin investigating healthy eating patterns, exploring different food grouping systems, and learning how to select a variety of foods that promote health. They should become acquainted with the variety of foods available, including foods from various cultures, and have opportunities to try foods that may not be a part of their regular diet. The concept that all foods have a place in a healthy diet should be emphasized. Although some foods provide more of the things the body needs than other foods, none have to be eliminated from a healthy diet except for medical or religious reasons. The *California Daily Food Guide* and the USDA food pyramid should be introduced and used to assist students in making healthy food choices.

Making healthy food choices

Grouping foods in many different ways—for example, by taste, smell, feel, color, sound, origin (plant or animal), or category

Establishing and maintaining healthy eating practices

Preparing and trying a variety of healthy foods, using safe and sanitary food preparation and storage techniques

Analyzing how food choices are influenced by peers, the media, the family, and the community

Physical activity:

Students should have opportunities to participate in enjoyable physical activities. As they enjoy movement, they can begin to develop an understanding of the means of achieving physical fitness. This understanding includes knowing the characteristics of a physically fit person and the physical, mental, emotional, and social benefits of regular physical activity.

Participating regularly in active play and a variety of enjoyable physical activities, with a focus on the pleasure of being active

Obtaining a sufficient amount of sleep

Observing safety rules during physical activities

Exploring ways to engage in enjoyable out-of-school play activities that promote fitness and health

Chapter 3
Health Education

III. Expectations
and Content,
by Grade Level

Kindergarten
Through
Grade Three

Unifying Idea:
Acceptance of personal
responsibility for
lifelong health

Expectation 1 (Continued)

Grade-level concepts and content	*Examples of skills and behaviors*
Mental and emotional health:	

As children explore the effects that eating nutritious foods and exercising sufficiently have on good health, they should learn that good health is a dynamic, unified state of physical, mental, emotional, and social well-being. A balanced routine of rest, work, play, and healthy food choices contributes to physical fitness and good health. In addition, fostering good family relationships and friendships and learning to base one's actions on personal values and ethical considerations promote mental and emotional health. The curriculum should, therefore, help students learn to balance self-interest with concern and caring for others.

Identifying and sharing feelings in appropriate ways

Demonstrating personal characteristics that contribute to self-confidence and self-esteem, such as honesty, integrity, respect for the dignity of others

Developing protective factors that help foster resiliency, such as participating in activities that promote positive bonding to peers and adults in the school and community and identifying a support system

Developing and using effective communication skills to enhance social interactions

Developing and using effective coping strategies, including critical thinking; effective decision making; goal setting; practice of problem solving, assertiveness, and refusal skills; and taking time for exercise and relaxation

Avoiding self-destructive behaviors and practicing self-control

Chapter 3
Health Education

III. Expectations
and Content,
by Grade Level

Kindergarten
Through
Grade Three

Unifying Idea:
Acceptance of personal
responsibility for
lifelong health

Expectation 2

Students will understand and demonstrate behaviors that prevent disease and speed recovery from illness.

Grade-level concepts and content	*Examples of skills and behaviors*

Disease prevention:

The curriculum should emphasize how behaviors can help prevent disease or reduce its influence. Students can explore ways in which communicable diseases are spread by pathogens. They should begin to understand that the risk of developing chronic diseases is influenced not only by one's behavior but also by environmental conditions and genetic predisposition. The content should include symptoms of major communicable diseases and the effect immunizations, health screenings, and sanitary practices can have on preventing the spread of diseases. Students can also investigate how faulty handling, storage, and preparation of food can produce food-borne illnesses.

Practicing good personal hygiene to prevent the spread of disease, such as washing one's hands and covering one's mouth when sneezing or coughing

Practicing positive health behaviors to reduce the risk of disease, such as:

1. Participating regularly in physical activities
2. Making healthy food choices
3. Acknowledging the importance of immunizations and demonstrating a willingness to cooperate in immunizations
4. Limiting exposure to communicable diseases as much as possible
5. Caring for wounds in a manner that supports healing

Cooperating in regular health screenings, including dental examinations

Preparing food in the classroom or school cafeteria as a way of learning about the importance of sanitary food preparation and storage to avoid communicable diseases and food-borne illnesses

**Kindergarten
Through
Grade Three**

Unifying Idea:
Acceptance of personal
responsibility for
lifelong health

Expectation 2 (Continued)

Grade-level concepts and content	*Examples of skills and behaviors*

Treatment of disease:

Students at this level should investigate the common symptoms of illness and recognize that being responsible for personal health also means alerting parents, guardians, or appropriate health-care personnel to any symptoms of disease. Students should explore how their behavior can help them recover from disease or manage its effects over the long term. Why medicines should be taken properly and why they should be taken only under the supervision of responsible adults should be emphasized.	Recognizing symptoms of common illnesses, such as fever, rashes, coughs, congestion, and wheezing, and describing them to parents or health-care providers Cooperating with parents and health-care providers in the treatment or management of disease, such as asthma Taking prescription or over-the-counter medicines properly under the direction of parents or health-care providers

Expectation 3

Students will practice behaviors that reduce the risk of becoming involved in potentially dangerous situations and react to potentially dangerous situations in ways that help to protect their health.

Potentially dangerous situations:

A key concept at this level is recognizing the potential for danger in everyday situations and behaving in ways that help to protect one's own safety and well-being. Students should be able to describe the characteristics of a safe environment and should be given opportunities to practice behaviors that promote a safe environment for themselves and others. The curriculum should include descriptions of potential dangers when students are in or near motor vehicles and when they are	Developing and using appropriate skills to identify, avoid when possible, and cope with potentially dangerous situations Practicing safe behavior in or near motorized vehicles, including crossing streets safely Practicing safe behavior in recreational activities, such as cycling and skating Practicing safe behavior in and near water Interacting safely with strangers

Chapter 3
Health Education

III. Expectations
and Content,
by Grade Level

**Kindergarten
Through
Grade Three**

Unifying Idea:
Acceptance of personal
responsibility for
lifelong health

Grade-level concepts and content	*Examples of skills and behaviors*

Potentially dangerous situations:

engaged in recreational activities, including references to drowning and falls. Students should know what to do if they become lost or separated from parents and should understand that they should never willingly go off with a stranger. They should be aware that being home alone is a big responsibility and is potentially dangerous. In addition, the curriculum should emphasize that young children should not handle firearms, which present a serious threat to the children's safety.	Developing and using appropriate skills to avoid, resolve, and cope with conflicts Reporting or obtaining assistance when faced with unsafe situations Practicing behaviors that help prevent poisonings, including learning never to smell, taste, or swallow unfamiliar items

Alcohol, tobacco, and other drugs:

Students should learn about the negative impact that chemical substances can have on health. The curriculum should discuss what drugs are, including alcohol, tobacco, and others, and describe the differences between helpful and potentially harmful substances. The concept of dependency should be introduced. And students should begin to learn to cope with an environment in which alcohol, tobacco, and other drugs are used and dependency exists by developing skills and behaviors that support positive health behaviors.	Exercising self-control Developing and using interpersonal and other communication skills Distinguishing between helpful and harmful substances Identifying ways to cope with or seek assistance as necessary when confronted with situations involving alcohol, tobacco, and other drugs

III. Expectations
and Content,
by Grade Level

**Kindergarten
Through
Grade Three**

Unifying Idea:
Acceptance of personal
responsibility for
lifelong health

Expectation 3 (Continued)

Grade-level concepts and content	*Examples of skills and behaviors*

Child abuse, including sexual exploitation:

After parents are notified and local standards are complied with, age-appropriate information about child abuse or neglect can be introduced. Included should be reference to each person's right to the privacy of his or her body and the appropriateness of telling others when touching is not welcome. Instruction should emphasize that a child is not at fault if the child is touched in an improper or uncomfortable way by an adult. The child's responsibility in this situation is to tell a trusted adult what had occurred.	Identifying ways to seek assistance if worried, abused, or threatened, including how to tell a trusted adult if uncomfortable touching occurs Developing and using communication skills to tell others when touching is unwanted

Emergencies:

Students should be taught appropriate ways to react during and after an emergency, including emergencies resulting from natural disasters, such as earthquakes. The first step is to recognize the seriousness of the situation. The second is to obtain assistance. Mitigating steps can substantially reduce health hazards resulting from natural disasters. Instruction should include descriptions of appropriate responses to fires and earthquakes and, depending on local needs, responses to such other potential disasters as floods. The role of adults in emergencies should be emphasized. For example, parents or teachers can help children. However, if they are not available, children should know how to seek help from other appropriate adults.	Recognizing emergencies and responding appropriately, including: 1. Knowing how to get out of the home in the event of a fire 2. Using a telephone appropriately to obtain help, including calling 911 if available 3. Providing name, address, and telephone number to a responsible adult 4. Knowing how to treat simple injuries, such as scratches, cuts, bruises, and first-degree burns 5. Practicing the stop, drop, and roll response to a clothing fire 6. Identifying and obtaining help from police officers, fire fighters, and medical personnel Practicing appropriate behavior during fire drills, earthquake drills, and other disaster drills

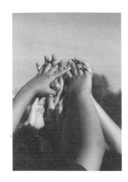

Unifying Idea
Respect for and promotion of the health of others

Expectations:

4. Students will understand and demonstrate how to play a positive, active role in promoting the health of their families.

5. Students will understand and demonstrate how to promote positive health practices within the school and community, including how to cultivate positive relationships with their peers.

Expectation 4

Students will understand and demonstrate how to play a positive, active role in promoting the health of their families.

Grade-level concepts and content	Examples of skills and behaviors
Roles of family members:	

Students should learn that a common trait of all successful families is a commitment to fostering the physical, mental, emotional, and social welfare of every member. Healthy people are actively and positively involved with their families.

Students should explore the role of parents and the extended family in supporting a strong family and promoting the health of children. For example, the limits parents set for children, the values or religious beliefs taught, and the behaviors and values modeled influence the behavior of children. Students can also explore the role of health-related rules in promoting the health of family members. For example, parents may require children to stay home when they have certain illnesses.

Students should explore the role of children in promoting the health

Supporting and valuing all family members

Demonstrating ways in which children can help support positive family interactions, such as listening to and following directions, following family rules, showing care and concern toward other family members, and interacting appropriately with family members

Developing and using effective communication skills, including nonviolent conflict resolution

Chapter 3
Health Education

III. Expectations
and Content,
by Grade Level

Kindergarten
Through
Grade Three

Unifying Idea:
Respect for and
promotion of the
health of others

Expectation 4 (Continued)

Grade-level concepts and content	Examples of skills and behaviors
Roles of family members:	
of the family and begin to develop the skills necessary to be a supportive family member.	
Change within the family:	
Such changes as pregnancy, birth, marriage, divorce or separation, illness, or death affect all family members and can generate strong emotions. Students should explore strategies for coping with change in the family.	Identifying feelings related to changes within the family and effectively expressing them to others in a positive way Using effective strategies to cope with change in the family, such as learning how to handle emotions by talking with a parent or other trusted adult about those feelings

Expectation 5

Students will understand and demonstrate how to promote positive health practices within the school and community, including how to cultivate positive relationships with their peers.

Friendship and peer relationships:

The curriculum should include an opportunity for students to examine how positive peer relationships contribute to good health. This exploration will help to lay the foundation for resisting negative peer pressure in later years. Students should explore the importance of having friends and the characteristics of good friends and begin to examine how others influence their behavior. They should also be helped to recognize that good communication is important for developing and maintaining friendships and should be guided to seek out healthy, positive friendships.	Knowing and using appropriate ways to make new friends Demonstrating acceptable methods of gaining attention Demonstrating acceptable ways to show or express feelings Demonstrating positive actions toward others, including acts of trust, kindness, respect, affection, listening, patience, and forgiveness and avoiding demeaning statements directed toward others Resolving conflicts in a positive, constructive way

Chapter 3
Health Education

III. Expectations
and Content,
by Grade Level

**Kindergarten
Through
Grade Three**

Unifying Idea:
Respect for and
promotion of the
health of others

Grade-level concepts and content	Examples of skills and behaviors

Friendship and peer relationships:

Students should also be encouraged to respect the dignity and worth of others, all of whom have special talents and abilities. Positive interactions are different from friendships, however. Although we may not like everyone with whom we interact, being able to communicate and work effectively with a variety of people is an important skill.

Violence is a public health issue. When conflicts cannot be resolved in a nonviolent manner, society suffers. Recognizing that there are positive ways to resolve conflict, students should begin to develop conflict-resolution skills at this time. They should learn a variety of strategies for handling negative feelings, including feelings of anger and disappointment.

School and community-based efforts to promote and protect health:

Students should understand why rules about health exist at home and at school and why students should respect those rules and encourage their friends and family members to do so as well. Students should be encouraged to assume responsibility for following the rules without being specifically reminded. In addition, the curriculum should include opportunities for students to develop an understanding of the way behavior affects the environment and participate in school or community efforts to support positive health behaviors. For example, students might examine sources of litter and determine ways to lessen the problem.

Understanding and following school rules related to health

Participating in school efforts to promote health—for example, a walk-a-thon, fund-raising events, or practices that support healthy food choices

Assuming responsibility for helping to take care of the school, such as picking up trash on the school grounds or helping other students assume responsibility for that action

Participating in community efforts to address local health and environmental issues—for example, recycling

Chapter 3
Health Education

III. Expectations
and Content,
by Grade Level

Kindergarten
Through
Grade Three

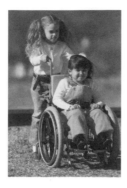

Unifying Idea

An understanding of the process of growth and development

Expectations:

6. Students will understand the variety of physical, mental, emotional, and social changes that occur throughout life.

7. Students will understand and accept individual differences in growth and development.

Expectation 6

Students will understand the variety of physical, mental, emotional, and social changes that occur throughout life.

Grade-level concepts and content	Examples of skills and behaviors
Life cycle:	
Students should learn that all living things come from other living things and have life cycles. For humans this process includes physical, mental, emotional, and social growth. Students should understand the stages of the life cycle from infancy to old age.	Describing the cycle of growth and development in humans and other animal species Demonstrating an understanding of the aging process, such as understanding why some older adults, including grandparents and great-grandparents, may have needs different from those of younger adults and children.

Expectation 7

Students will understand and accept individual differences in growth and development.

Growth and development:	
Students should explore the universal aspects of growth. However, they should also recognize that each individual has a unique pattern of growth and development. The major factors that determine individual differences, especially in height and weight, should be	Demonstrating an understanding of individual differences, such as differences in appearance or learning styles, through positive, constructive actions

Grade-level concepts and content	*Examples of skills and behaviors*

Growth and development:

highlighted, including genetics and dietary and exercise habits. Although persons with disabilities are different from others, they are not inferior. Students should be encouraged to accept those with disabilities. They should try to walk in the shoes of a person with special needs and determine how they would like people to treat them if they had disabilities.	Adapting group activities to include a variety of students—for example, blind students or students in wheelchairs

Mental and emotional development:

Students should explore the mental and emotional aspects of growth and development. For example, they should learn that many of the emotions they experience throughout life are also felt by other people. When feeling sad, angry, or confused, they will find that talking about feelings with a parent, trusted peer, or other adult is an appropriate coping skill.	Identifying, expressing, and managing feelings appropriately Developing and using effective communication skills

Chapter 3
Health Education

III. Expectations
and Content,
by Grade Level

**Kindergarten
Through
Grade Three**

Unifying Idea:
An understanding of
the process of growth
and development

Chapter 3
Health Education

III. Expectations
and Content,
by Grade Level

Kindergarten
Through
Grade Three

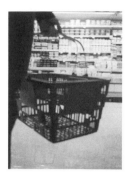

Unifying Idea
Informed use of health-related information, products, and services

Expectation:

8. Students will identify information, products, and services that may be helpful or harmful to their health.

Expectation 8

Students will identify information, products, and services that may be helpful or harmful to their health.

Grade-level concepts and content	*Examples of skills and behaviors*
Products and services:	
Students should begin to explore how the health-care system functions by identifying places for obtaining health services and learning what specific services are offered. They should identify types of health-care workers and persons qualified to provide health advice and care, thereby laying the groundwork for a discussion of health quackery in later years. They should also explore sources of health-related information and products. Students at this grade span should begin to recognize that they are consumers and that consumer decisions are influenced by a variety of factors. They should begin to explore the advertising strategies used to influence the selection and use of health-related products and services as well as the use of alcohol and tobacco.	Identifying places for obtaining health and social services and learning what types of services are provided

Identifying health-care workers

Identifying a variety of consumer influences and analyzing how those influences affect decisions |

Grade-level concepts and content	Examples of skills and behaviors

Food choices:

Students should explore how family, school, friends, the community, advertising, and the food industry all play a role in influencing what children prefer to eat, what is available for them to eat, and what their eating environments are like. Students should recognize that all of these factors influence the food choices they make.

Students should explore sources of nutrition information and recognize that food labels are a convenient and important source for this information. They should learn how to identify the contents of packaged foods and begin to learn how to use labels to compare food products.

Reading and interpreting some of the information available on food labels, such as identifying sugar, salt, and fat as ingredients

Using labels to compare the contents of food products

Identifying ads and recognizing strategies used to influence decisions

Practicing various positive responses to those influences

Chapter 3
Health Education

III. Expectations and Content, by Grade Level

Kindergarten Through Grade Three

Unifying Idea:
Informed use of health-related information, products, and services

Grades Four Through Six

Students in grades four through six are assuming more responsibility for their own health and well-being. They can benefit from instruction that fosters the development of positive health behaviors and prevention of negative, unhealthy behaviors. Particularly important in the middle grades is the onset of adolescence, which can begin as early as third grade for some students. Others will develop more slowly. Students at this level begin to become acutely aware of their physical development and the varying rates of development among their peers. In addition, children's orientation to the peer group tends to increase during this age span. Most children experience a growing need to be and feel normal at precisely the time when growth and development vary widely even within the same classroom. Many students are also likely to feel pressure to act grown-up by experimenting with alcohol, tobacco, or other drugs. Acceptance of differences in individual growth and development as well as strategies to prevent the use of alcohol, tobacco, and other drugs need to be woven throughout the curriculum at this time.

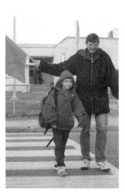

Unifying Idea
Acceptance of personal responsibility for lifelong health

Expectations:

1. Students will demonstrate ways in which they can enhance and maintain their health and well-being.
2. Students will understand and demonstrate behaviors that prevent disease and speed recovery from illness.
3. Students will practice behaviors that reduce the risk of becoming involved in potentially dangerous situations and react to potentially dangerous situations in ways that help to protect their health.

Expectation 1

Students will demonstrate ways in which they can enhance and maintain their health and well-being.

Grade-level concepts and content	*Examples of skills and behaviors*
The human body:	
As students assume responsibility for personal care and self-grooming, they should continue to explore the link between their behavior and	■ Practicing good personal hygiene, with particular attention to the changing needs of preadolescents and adolescents

■ Identifies previously introduced skills or behaviors that should be built on and reinforced.

Chapter 3
Health Education

III. Expectations
and Content,
by Grade Level

**Grades Four
Through Six**

Unifying Idea:
Acceptance of personal
responsibility for
lifelong health

Grade-level concepts and content	*Examples of skills and behaviors*

The human body:

health. For example, as puberty begins, behavioral changes related to personal health habits may be involved for some students.

The curriculum at this level should also include more in-depth information about body systems and their relation to personal health. Students should learn how body systems are interrelated, how they function to fight disease, and how they are influenced by environmental conditions.

■ Using protective equipment, such as a helmet when cycling, or practicing behaviors to protect the body, such as applying sunscreen when appropriate

Food choices:

Building on the concepts and skills learned at the kindergarten through grade three level, students should continue to explore how food choices can affect their health and well-being. They should continue to learn about food classification systems and begin to learn about the nutrients in foods. *The California Daily Food Guide* and the USDA food pyramid should be used to assist students in making healthy food choices from a variety of ethnic cuisines. The effects food choices have on body composition and optimal health should be explored as well as the dangers of eating disorders. Students should examine how food-preparation methods and food-handling practices affect the safety and nutrient quality of foods.

■ Making healthy food choices, with emphasis on:
  1. Basing decisions upon nutrient content
  2. Selecting foods that promote oral health

■ Establishing and maintaining healthy eating practices

■ Preparing a variety of healthy foods, using safe and sanitary food preparation and storage techniques, with an emphasis on how food-handling and preparation practices affect the safety and nutrient quality of foods

■ Analyzing how food choices are influenced

Practicing kitchen safety, such as using knives, stoves, and ovens correctly and carefully

■ Identifies previously introduced skills or behaviors that should be built on and reinforced.

III. Expectations
and Content,
by Grade Level

**Grades Four
Through Six**

Unifying Idea:
Acceptance of personal
responsibility for
lifelong health

Expectation 1 (Continued)

Grade-level concepts and content	*Examples of skills and behaviors*
Physical activity:	
Students should continue to enjoy physical activities and should learn to set and use personal goals for developing or maintaining physical fitness, recognizing that even moderate regular activity can help prevent obesity and heart disease. Students should also investigate the relationships involving aerobic endurance, body composition, flexibility, muscular strength and endurance, and self-image.	▪ Obtaining a sufficient amount of sleep ▪ Observing safety rules during physical activities ▪ Exploring ways to engage in enjoyable out-of-school play activities that promote fitness and health Participating regularly in a variety of enjoyable physical activities that promote aerobic conditioning, flexibility, and muscular strength and endurance both inside and outside of school Setting personal fitness goals Monitoring progress toward meeting fitness goals
Mental and emotional health:	
Mental and emotional health, like physical fitness, can be cultivated and enhanced. Students in grades three through six have an increasing sensitivity to peer influence and feel acutely the need to belong to a group. The curriculum should continue to include opportunities for students to identify and seek protective factors that help foster resiliency. Students should learn that although preadolescence and adolescence are frequently periods of emotional turmoil, various coping strategies can be used to overcome feelings of inadequacy and depression.	▪ Identifying and sharing feelings in appropriate ways ▪ Demonstrating personal characteristics that contribute to self-confidence and self-esteem, such as honesty, integrity, respect for the dignity of others ▪ Developing protective factors that help foster resiliency, such as participating in activities that promote positive bonding to peers and adults in the school and the community ▪ Developing and using effective communication skills

▪ Identifies previously introduced skills or behaviors that should be built on and reinforced.

Chapter 3
Health Education

III. Expectations
and Content,
by Grade Level

**Grades Four
Through Six**

Unifying Idea:
Acceptance of personal
responsibility for
lifelong health

Grade-level concepts and content	*Examples of skills and behaviors*

Mental and emotional health:

High self-esteem and a sense of optimism and control over one's life are linked to one's success as a happy, productive human being. Students should have opportunities to bond to the school and community and to receive positive recognition for success. This age level is appropriate for introducing students to the effects of stress, including a discussion of what causes stress and how it can be detrimental to health unless various coping strategies are used to deal with it.

- Developing and using effective coping strategies, including critical thinking, effective decision making, goal setting, and problem solving; practicing assertiveness and refusal skills; and taking time for exercise and relaxation

- Avoiding self-destructive behaviors

Practicing strategies for resisting negative peer pressure

Expectation 2

Students will understand and demonstrate behaviors that prevent disease and speed recovery from illness.

Disease prevention:

A wide range of communicable and chronic diseases, including genetic disorders, should be the focus of the curriculum for this outcome at this grade span. Students should develop an understanding of the difference between communicable and noncommunicable diseases. Causes of diseases and the role of positive health practices (e.g., regular medical and dental examinations, immunizations, aerobic exercise, proper nutrition) in avoiding, delaying, or minimizing the onset of diseases should also be emphasized. The curriculum should investigate how people with diseases

- Practicing good personal hygiene to prevent the spread of disease

- Practicing positive health behaviors to reduce the risk of disease

- Cooperating in regular health screenings, including dental examinations

Demonstrating safe care and concern toward ill persons in the family, the school, and the community

■ Identifies previously introduced skills or behaviors that should be built on and reinforced.

Chapter 3
Health Education

III. Expectations
and Content,
by Grade Level

Grades Four
Through Six

Unifying Idea:
Acceptance of personal
responsibility for
lifelong health

Expectation 2 (Continued)

Grade-level concepts and content	Examples of skills and behaviors

Disease prevention:

are treated, including how prejudice and ignorance can lead to discrimination against persons with diseases or chronic conditions.	

Treatment of disease:

As students take more responsibility for their health, they develop a deeper understanding of the need to follow prescribed health-care procedures and cooperate with parents and health-care providers to facilitate recovery from disease when possible or to enhance long-term management of chronic diseases. The treatment or management of the major communicable and chronic diseases should be presented, including scientific contributions that have helped to protect people from disease and disorders. Students who have health problems or chronic conditions should begin to accept responsibility for their role in treatment, including the proper use of medication. The effects of family and cultural influences on the care of disease and the usefulness of participating in support groups or activities should also be explored.

■ Recognizing symptoms of common illnesses

■ Cooperating in treatment or management of disease, with an emphasis on accepting responsibility for such cooperation and communicating appropriately with parents and health-care providers

■ Taking prescription and over-the-counter medicines properly; never taking medicine prescribed for someone else

Interpreting correctly instructions for taking medicine

■ Identifies previously introduced skills or behaviors that should be built on and reinforced.

Chapter 3
Health Education

III. Expectations
and Content,
by Grade Level

**Grades Four
Through Six**

Unifying Idea:
Acceptance of personal
responsibility for
lifelong health

Expectation 3

Students will practice behaviors that reduce the risk of becoming involved in potentially dangerous situations and react to potentially dangerous situations in ways that help to protect their health.

Grade-level concepts and content	*Examples of skills and behaviors*

Potentially dangerous situations:

At this level students should learn that some potentially dangerous situations can be handled through routine safety precautions, including behaving appropriately in or near motor vehicles; observing safe play and exercise practices; identifying hazards in the home, school, and community; and participating in activities to remove hazards.

Students should understand how to minimize the potential for injury when interacting with others who exhibit dangerous behavior. For example, one option is to leave the situation or, if appropriate, encourage the individual to stop the dangerous behavior. Conflict-resolution skills should be further refined and practiced.

■ Developing and using appropriate skills to identify, avoid when possible, and cope with potentially dangerous situations

■ Practicing safe behavior in and near motorized vehicles

■ Practicing safe behavior in recreational activities

■ Practicing safe behavior in and near water

■ Developing and using appropriate skills to avoid, resolve, and cope with conflicts, emphasizing how peers can help each other avoid and cope with conflict

■ Reporting or obtaining assistance when faced with unsafe situations

Understanding and following rules prohibiting possession of weapons at school

Alcohol, tobacco, and other drugs:

Because experimentation with alcohol, tobacco, or other drugs often begins in the upper elementary grades, students should develop the knowledge, skills, and strategies for choosing not to use a wide range of harmful chemical substances. They should learn ways to identify drugs; the effects of drugs on different parts

■ Exercising self-control

■ Developing and using interpersonal and other communication skills, such as assertiveness, refusal, negotiation, and conflict-resolution skills, to avoid use of alcohol, tobacco, and other drugs

■ Distinguishing between helpful and harmful substances

■ Identifies previously introduced skills or behaviors that should be built on and reinforced.

Chapter 3
Health Education

III. Expectations
and Content,
by Grade Level

Grades Four
Through Six

Unifying Idea:
Acceptance of personal
responsibility for
lifelong health

Expectation 3 (Continued)

Grade-level concepts and content	*Examples of skills and behaviors*

Alcohol, tobacco, and other drugs:

of the body; the reasons for not using specific substances; and the effects and consequences of use. In addition, they should learn the school rules prohibiting the use of alcohol, tobacco, and other drugs and should be aware that these substances are illegal for minors or all persons. Students should understand the influences that promote drug use and develop the skills necessary to resist those influences; know how and where to obtain help when confronted with potentially dangerous or harmful situations involving chemical substances; and make a commitment not to use or distribute alcohol, tobacco, or other drugs.

■ Identifying ways to cope with or seek assistance as necessary when confronted with situations involving alcohol, tobacco, or other drugs

Differentiating between the use and misuse of prescription and nonprescription drugs

Avoiding, recognizing, and responding to negative social influences and pressure to use alcohol, tobacco, or other drugs

Using positive peer pressure to help counteract the negative effects of living in an environment where alcohol, tobacco, or other drug abuse or dependency exists

Identifying ways of obtaining help to resist pressure to use alcohol, tobacco, or other drugs

Child abuse, including sexual exploitation:

Students should be aware that no one, not even a parent, has the right to abuse a child or another family member physically. Neglect and child abuse are serious problems that may require outside assistance.

After parents are notified, the strategies presented in discussions of alcohol, tobacco, and other drugs can be expanded to help students learn how to resist pressure to become sexually active and where to seek help or advice if needed. Information on how to resist sexual abuse or exploitation should also be presented.

■ Identifying ways to seek assistance if concerned, abused, or threatened, including how to overcome fear of telling

Recognizing and avoiding situations that can increase risk of abuse, such as leaning into a car when giving directions to a stranger

■ Identifies previously introduced skills or behaviors that should be built on and reinforced.

Grade-level concepts and content	Examples of skills and behaviors

Emergencies:

Building on earlier instruction in proper responses to natural disasters, students should have the opportunity to learn and demonstrate emergency preparation procedures and proficiency in basic first-aid procedures, including proper response to breathing and choking problems, bleeding, shock, poisonings, and minor burns. Older students can also learn cardiopulmonary resuscitation, in addition to basic first aid, if taught by certified instructors.

Recognizing emergencies and responding appropriately, including:

1. Knowing where to find emergency supplies, such as a flashlight and a first-aid kit
2. Demonstrating proficiency in basic first-aid procedures, such as proper response to breathing and choking problems, bleeding, shock, poisonings, and minor burns
3. Using universal precautions when dealing with other people's blood

Understanding the family emergency plan and developing the skills necessary to follow the plan

Chapter 3
Health Education

III. Expectations and Content, by Grade Level

Grades Four Through Six

Unifying Idea:
Acceptance of personal responsibility for lifelong health

Chapter 3
Health Education

III. Expectations
and Content,
by Grade Level

Grades Four
Through Six

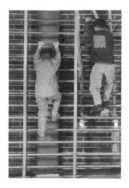

Unifying Idea
Respect for and promotion of the health of others

Expectations:

4. Students will understand and demonstrate how to play a positive, active role in promoting the health of their families.

5. Students will understand and demonstrate how to promote positive health practices within the school and community, including how to cultivate positive relationships with their peers.

Expectation 4

Students will understand and demonstrate how to play a positive, active role in promoting the health of their families.

Grade-level concepts and content	Examples of skills and behaviors
Roles of family members:	
Building on the concept of the family as a major source of a person's health, students should recognize that because the roles of children change as they mature, parents may have different expectations of children versus adolescents. Students should explore ways in which they can contribute to their family, including participating in family activities, practicing health-promoting behaviors with the family, and assuming more responsibility for household tasks.	■ Supporting and valuing all family members ■ Demonstrating ways in which children can help support positive family interactions ■ Developing and using effective communication skills Practicing health-promoting behaviors with the family, such as encouraging family walks and meals at which the entire family is present Participating in daily activities that help maintain the family
Change within the family:	
Changes within and outside the family may affect both individuals and family members. Students at this grade level should have the opportunity to examine the effects of change on the family and develop	■ Identifying feelings related to changes within the family and effectively expressing them to others in a positive way

■ Identifies previously introduced skills or behaviors that should be built on and reinforced.

Grade-level concepts and content	Examples of skills and behaviors

Change within the family:

coping strategies to deal with changes when they occur. The important point to consider is that although families are challenged by such events as a serious illness or divorce, families can and do cope and may in fact grow stronger as a result of the challenge. Good communication in a family is a key coping skill, and positive ways to resolve conflict should continue to be addressed. Students should be able to identify community resources that provide help to families with problems.

■ Using effective strategies to cope with change in the family, including identifying a support system

Chapter 3
Health Education

III. Expectations and Content, by Grade Level

Grades Four Through Six

Unifying Idea:
Respect for and promotion of the health of others

Expectation 5

Students will understand and demonstrate how to promote positive health practices within the school and community, including how to cultivate positive relationships with their peers.

Friendship and peer relationships:

Students should explore how people can play active roles in promoting healthy relationships with peers. They should be aware that peer influence has the potential to be either positive or negative. Students should be encouraged to seek opportunities to be a positive role model.

■ Knowing and using appropriate ways to make new friends

■ Demonstrating acceptable methods of gaining attention

■ Demonstrating acceptable ways to show or express feelings

■ Demonstrating positive actions toward others

■ Resolving conflicts in a positive, constructive way

Demonstrating how to resist negative peer pressure

■ Identifies previously introduced skills or behaviors that should be built on and reinforced.

Chapter 3
Health Education

III. Expectations
and Content,
by Grade Level

**Grades Four
Through Six**

Unifying Idea:
Respect for and
promotion of the
health of others

Expectation 5 (Continued)

Grade-level concepts and content	*Examples of skills and behaviors*

School and community-based efforts to promote and protect health:

Students should explore how their school promotes and protects the health of students. For example, students should examine school policies related to health, nutrition, and safety and understand the reasons for those policies. They should understand that by following the policies, they are helping to promote health at school. Further, students should explore how people can play active roles in the school and community to promote health and should have opportunities to participate in positive health practices in school and community settings.

They should begin to explore the role of the health department and other community health and social service agencies in health promotion and disease prevention. Local, state, and national laws and regulations that promote public health and the safety of the community should be identified and examined, including those designed to protect the environment. Recycling, developing safe and adequate food supplies and environmentally safe food packaging, and dealing with hunger and food waste within their communities should be introduced. Students should investigate ways in which they can participate in or enhance school and community efforts to promote health.

■ Understanding and following school rules related to health

■ Participating in school efforts to promote health; for example, helping to select fund-raising activities that are consistent with efforts to promote health, such as choosing a jog-a-thon rather than a candy sale

■ Assuming responsibility for helping to take care of the school, such as picking up trash on the school grounds and helping other students assume responsibility for that action

■ Participating in community efforts to address local health and environmental issues

Contributing to the strengthening of health-related policies at school, such as serving on a student safety committee

Recognizing that public policies and laws influence health-related issues

■ Identifies previously introduced skills or behaviors that should be built on and reinforced.

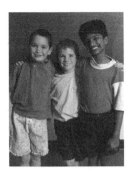

Unifying Idea
An understanding of the process of growth and development

Expectations:

6. Students will understand the variety of physical, mental, emotional, and social changes that occur throughout life.

7. Students will understand and accept individual differences in growth and development.

Chapter 3
Health Education

III. Expectations
and Content,
by Grade Level

**Grades Four
Through Six**

Expectation 6

Students will understand the variety of physical, mental, emotional, and social changes that occur throughout life.

Grade-level concepts and content	Examples of skills and behaviors
Life cycle:	

Note: The *Education Code* requires parental notification before discussion of human reproductive organs and their functions and processes. Students at this level are beginning to enter puberty and are curious, perhaps concerned, about the physical changes they are experiencing. Instruction should emphasize that all people are sexual beings and that it is natural for preadolescents and adolescents to want to understand human sexuality. The curriculum should help students understand the human reproductive process and the physical, mental, emotional, and social changes that occur during puberty. To be included are descriptions of sexual maturation, acne, changes in voice, growth of body and facial hair, menstruation, and sperm development. As they reach puberty, students should be made	Recognizing the changes that occur during preadolescence Using correct terminology for body parts Practicing good personal hygiene, paying particular attention to the changing needs of preadolescents and adolescents Recognizing emotions Managing feelings appropriately, including being able to express feelings and practice self-control Developing and using effective communication skills to discuss with parents or other trusted adults the changes that occur during preadolescence

Chapter 3
Health Education

III. Expectations
and Content,
by Grade Level

**Grades Four
Through Six**

Unifying Idea:
An understanding of
the process of growth
and development

Expectation 6 (Continued)

Grade-level concepts and content	*Examples of skills and behaviors*
Life cycle:	
aware of toxic shock syndrome (TSS), its symptoms, and the means of preventing it. Also important are the social and emotional changes of adolescence—for example, a growing sensitivity to peer influence, family tensions, and mood swings. Cognitive and intellectual development should also be considered. Students should be encouraged to talk to their parents or other responsible adults if they have questions about sexuality or puberty and related changes.	

Expectation 7

Students will understand and accept individual differences in growth and development.

Growth and development:	
The rate of change during puberty varies with each person. Students should be encouraged to be comfortable with their own progress and to like and accept themselves. The curriculum should emphasize that there is no perfect body type and that people vary widely in size, height, shape, and rate of maturation.	■ Demonstrating an understanding of individual differences ■ Adapting group activities to include a variety of students Developing a realistic body image Recognizing problems associated with not having a realistic body image, including dieting and eating disorders, and seeking appropriate help
Mental and emotional development:	
Students should continue to explore the mental and emotional aspects of growing and developing.	■ Identifying, expressing, and managing feelings appropriately

■ Identifies previously introduced skills or behaviors that should be built on and reinforced.

95

Chapter 3
Health Education

III. Expectations
and Content,
by Grade Level

Grades Four
Through Six

Grade-level concepts and content	*Examples of skills and behaviors*

Mental and emotional development:

They should be encouraged to focus on the future and develop strategies for coping with the changes of adolescence. Instruction should emphasize understanding differences, including individuals' unique strengths and weaknesses and the ways in which students can support each other in facing the uncertainties of adolescence. It is especially important at this time, when many students begin to be more group-oriented, to emphasize the need to include all students, especially those with disabilities and special needs.

■ Developing and using effective communication skills

Recognizing one's own strengths and limitations

Developing and using coping strategies, including critical thinking, effective decision making, goal setting, and problem solving; developing assertiveness and refusal skills; and taking time for exercise and relaxation

Developing a focus on the future, such as having realistic short-term and long-term goals and delaying gratification

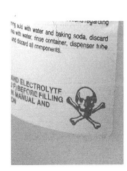

Unifying Idea
Informed use of health-related information, products, and services

Expectation:

8. Students will identify information, products, and services that may be helpful or harmful to their health.

Expectation 8

Students will identify information, products, and services that may be helpful or harmful to their health.

Grade-level concepts and content	*Examples of skills and behaviors*

Products and services:

Students at this level should begin to identify the range of health services in the community and explore how their families can access

■ Identifying places for obtaining health and social services and knowing what types of services are provided

■ Identifies previously introduced skills or behaviors that should be built on and reinforced.

Chapter 3
Health Education

III. Expectations
and Content,
by Grade Level

Grades Four
Through Six

Unifying Idea:
Informed use of
health-related
information,
products,
and services

Expectation 8 (Continued)

Grade-level concepts and content	Examples of skills and behaviors

Products and services:

needed services, including developing the ability to distinguish between situations that require health services and those that do not. An examination of community health services can be linked to an exploration of health-related careers, including careers related to food preparation and food service.

Consumer health care products are another important focus of the curriculum at this level. Students should be able to distinguish products and services that are necessary, those that are not necessary, and those that may be harmful. Characteristics of health care quackery should be presented. To be included is the idea that quackery is more likely to flourish in those areas of health—pain management, beauty aids, weight control, cancer treatment—where standard medicine is least successful or when expectations are unrealistic. Students should look critically at health claims and the factors that influence the selection of products and services, including ways in which advertising and peer pressure can influence students' images of themselves.

■ Identifying health-care workers

■ Identifying a variety of consumer influences and analyzing how those influences affect decisions

Recognizing helpful products and services

Using critical-thinking skills to analyze marketing and advertising techniques and their influence on the selection of health-related services and products

Seeking care from the school nurse or school-linked services together with their families when appropriate, such as when needed for proper management of asthma

Discussing home care with parents when appropriate

Food choices:

As students mature, they become increasingly more responsible for their own health and have greater

■ Reading and interpreting the information available on food labels, such as the amount of sugar, salt, or fat contained in the food

■ Identifies previously introduced skills or behaviors that should be built on and reinforced.

Chapter 3
Health Education

III. Expectations
and Content,
by Grade Level

**Grades Four
Through Six**

Unifying Idea:
Informed use of
health-related
information,
products,
and services

Grade-level concepts and content	*Examples of skills and behaviors*

Food choices:

opportunities to purchase and prepare their own food. Thus, the need for good consumer skills increases. Students should explore the influence of self-image, peer influences, and advertising on food choices. They should learn to use all the information on food labels when making decisions about which foods to buy and should have opportunities to learn basic food-preparation and handling techniques.

Because of their growing independence, many students have more frequent opportunities to eat away from home. As a result they have opportunities to try new foods and practice ways to maintain a nutritionally balanced diet. The curriculum should include ways to make food choices in a variety of eating environments, including fast-food outlets. As their circle of friends expands, students will have greater exposure to differing family customs, backgrounds, and eating patterns. This is an opportune time to explore a variety of ethnic and cultural foods, food patterns, and customs, using both the classroom and the school cafeteria.

- Using labels to compare the contents of food products, including a comparison of the cost of various foods according to their nutritional value

Using critical-thinking skills to analyze marketing and advertising techniques and their influence on food selection

Using valid nutrition information to make healthy food choices

Purchasing nutritious foods in a variety of settings

Using unit pricing to determine the most economical purchases

Analyzing and tasting foods from different ethnic and cultural groups

Developing basic food-preparation skills, including safe and sanitary food preparation and storage

- Identifies previously introduced skills or behaviors that should be built on and reinforced.

Middle School

Students in middle school are becoming more independent of their parents and increasingly more subject to peer approval than are younger children. They are concerned, at times preoccupied, with changes in their bodies and they often begin to focus on themselves and to be critical of themselves and others. Able to understand that certain behaviors have undesirable consequences, they may have difficulty in accepting that such consequences could happen to them. An awareness of immediate consequences (for example, bad breath as a result of smoking) rather than long-term consequences is more likely to motivate students. The curriculum for this grade span focuses in part on the personal health habits appropriate to the changing needs of adolescents. But students should also continue to explore and practice the skills necessary for developing lifelong positive health habits. Although prevention remains the mainstay of the curriculum at this level, additional elements are the early identification of health problems and appropriate intervention. Students should always be encouraged to discuss personal and health problems with their parents or guardians. Information about local resources for health-related support and assistance should also be provided as part of the curriculum.

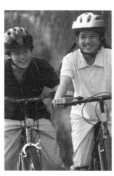

Unifying Idea
Acceptance of personal responsibility for lifelong health

Expectations:

1. Students will demonstrate ways in which they can enhance and maintain their health and well-being.
2. Students will understand and demonstrate behaviors that prevent disease and speed recovery from illness.
3. Students will practice behaviors that reduce the risk of becoming involved in potentially dangerous situations and react to potentially dangerous situations in ways that help to protect their health.

Expectation 1

Students will demonstrate ways in which they can enhance and maintain their health and well-being.

Chapter 3
Health Education

III. Expectations
and Content,
by Grade Level

Middle School

Unifying Idea:
Acceptance of personal
responsibility for
lifelong health

Grade-level concepts and content	*Examples of skills and behaviors*
The human body:	

The immediate and long-term effects of personal health habits on body systems are appropriate areas of study for this grade span. For example, students might explore the short-term and long-term effects of a high-fat diet and a sedentary lifestyle on the cardiovascular system. They should continue to examine how body systems are interconnected and how the immune system prevents or combats disease. Because environmental conditions also affect body systems, students should be able to demonstrate ways to protect themselves from exposure to conditions that are potentially harmful.

As they continue to explore the unifying idea of acceptance of personal responsibility and the human body, students continue to recognize that a perfect body type does not exist and that people vary widely in size, height, shape, and rate of maturation. They should be encouraged to be comfortable with their own progress and to like and accept themselves.

■ Practicing good personal hygiene, including accepting responsibility for making those behaviors part of a normal routine

■ Recognizing and avoiding when possible, environmental conditions that are potentially harmful, such as exposure to pesticides or lead paint

■ Using protective equipment, such as goggles to protect the eyes when appropriate, or practicing behaviors to protect the body, such as applying sunscreen, exercising, or making healthy food choices

Recognizing and accepting differences in body types and maturation levels

Food choices:

Students should be encouraged to develop a personal nutrition plan based on food choices and calorie levels that promotes health and reduces the risk of disease. They

■ Making healthy food choices in a variety of settings, including the selection of foods according to calculated energy expenditure and healthy body composition

■ Identifies previously introduced skills or behaviors that should be built on and reinforced.

III. Expectations
and Content,
by Grade Level

Middle School

Unifying Idea:
Acceptance of personal
responsibility for
lifelong health

Expectation 1 (Continued)

Grade-level concepts and content	*Examples of skills and behaviors*
Food choices:	
should continue to explore the wide variety of healthy food choices available in all cultures and should have opportunities to taste and prepare low-cost foods and favorite foods in ways that make those foods healthy choices. The content should include the interrelationships among total calories, food sources of calories, energy expenditure, and body composition. Because adolescents have unique nutritional needs, they should understand that the variety and quantity of food they eat can influence their growth and development. Further, they should examine how their food choices are influenced by their own emotions and by other sources, such as their peers or the media.	■ Establishing and maintaining healthy eating practices ■ Preparing a variety of healthy foods, using safe food preparation and storage techniques ■ Analyzing how food choices are influenced Comparing caloric values of foods according to the percentage of fat, protein, and carbohydrate they contain Selecting appropriate practices to maintain, lose, or gain weight according to individual needs and scientific research
Physical activity:	
Students should be made aware of the importance of variety and enjoyment in maintaining an exercise program and should have opportunities to participate regularly in a variety of physical activities at school and outside school. In addition, they should continue to set personal goals for developing or maintaining physical fitness. They should look for opportunities to set up a personal fitness program because a physically active lifestyle contributes to their personal health. They should examine the influence of frequency, intensity, duration, and type of physical	■ Obtaining a sufficient amount of sleep ■ Observing safety rules during physical activities ■ Exploring ways to engage in out-of-school activities that promote fitness and health ■ Participating regularly in a variety of enjoyable physical activities ■ Developing and initiating a personal fitness plan that includes setting fitness goals and monitoring progress toward meeting those goals

■ Identifies previously introduced skills or behaviors that should be built on and reinforced.

Chapter 3
Health Education

III. Expectations
and Content,
by Grade Level

Middle School

Unifying Idea:
Acceptance of personal
responsibility for
lifelong health

Grade-level concepts and content	*Examples of skills and behaviors*

Physical activity:

activity on aerobic endurance, body composition, flexibility, and muscular strength and endurance. Finally, they should analyze ways in which physical activity contributes to physical, mental, emotional, and social health.

Mental and emotional health:

Students' explorations of the mental and emotional aspects of health should build on those examined at earlier grade levels. Particular emphasis should be placed on emotional development during adolescence, including an examination of mood swings, depression, and suicide. Students should understand that seeking assistance for mental and emotional problems is appropriate and should have opportunities to develop the skills needed to seek assistance. The positive aspects of mental and emotional health, such as friendship, continue to be of great importance and should also receive attention in the curriculum. In addition, students should continue to explore the connections between physical, mental, emotional, and social health and should be encouraged to pursue leisure-time activities that promote that health.

The curriculum should provide opportunities for all students to feel valued and have experiences that foster positive bonding to their

- Demonstrating personal characteristics that contribute to self-confidence and self-esteem, such as honesty, integrity, responsibility, and respecting the dignity of others

- Developing protective factors that help foster resiliency, such as participating in activities that promote positive bonding to peers and adults in the school and community, and developing and maintaining a focus on the future

- Developing and using effective communication skills

- Developing and using effective coping strategies, emphasizing strategies for coping with feelings of inadequacy, sadness, and depression. Examples include talking over problems with parents or religious leaders, understanding that feelings of isolation and depression will pass, examining the situation leading to the feelings, seeking appropriate assistance if depression persists, obtaining

- Identifies previously introduced skills or behaviors that should be built on and reinforced.

Chapter 3
Health Education

III. Expectations
and Content,
by Grade Level

Middle School

Unifying Idea:
Acceptance of personal
responsibility for
lifelong health

Expectation 1 (Continued)

Grade-level concepts and content	*Examples of skills and behaviors*
Mental and emotional health:	

peers, school, and community. These experiences are especially important for students at higher risk of suicide because these students thereby learn to cope with feelings of isolation, inadequacy, sadness, and depression and begin to overcome those feelings. Strategies that can be explored to help students cope with those feelings include talking over problems, understanding that feelings of isolation and depression will pass, examining the situation leading to the feelings, seeking appropriate assistance if depression persists, obtaining medical treatment for organically caused depression, and participating in regular aerobic exercise.

appropriate health care for depression, and participating in regular aerobic exercise

■ Avoiding self-destructive behaviors

■ Practicing strategies for resisting negative peer pressure

Identifying the strongest risk factors for negative behaviors in their own lives and developing effective strategies for counteracting the effect of these risk factors

Managing strong feelings and boredom

Selecting entertainment that promotes mental and physical health

Expectation 2

Students will understand and demonstrate behaviors that prevent disease and speed recovery from illness.

Disease prevention:

Students should acquire the knowledge and skills needed to develop a personal action plan for the prevention or early detection of disease.

Students should focus on the major chronic and communicable diseases prevalent at different stages of life, analyzing risks for contracting specific diseases based on pathogenic, genetic, environmental, and behavioral factors. They should continue

■ Practicing good personal hygiene to prevent the spread of disease

■ Practicing positive health behaviors to reduce the risk of disease

■ Cooperating in regular health screenings, including dental examinations

■ Safely demonstrating care and concern toward ill persons in the family, the school, and the community

■ Identifies previously introduced skills or behaviors that should be built on and reinforced.

Grade-level concepts and content	Examples of skills and behaviors

Disease prevention:

to explore how positive health practices, such as aerobic exercise and proper nutrition, influence the risk and severity of disease. They should also learn how common behavioral disorders contribute to chronic conditions, perhaps studying anorexia nervosa and its complications. They should begin to learn self-exam procedures and understand the role of self-examination in early detection of disease. In addition to learning how to prevent and cope with diseases in themselves, students should learn that people with diseases need the support and compassion of others.

The prevention of sexually transmitted diseases (STDs), especially HIV/AIDS, should be emphasized at this grade span but only after consideration of *Education Code* mandates (see Appendix A). Students should be able to describe the causes of HIV infection and other sexually transmitted diseases as well as modes of transmission, symptoms, effects, and methods of prevention.

A strong emphasis should be placed on abstinence from sexual activity and safer sexual practices for those youths who are sexually active. However, sexual activity ("safe sex") is not being advocated. Abstinence from sexual activity is the only totally effective way to avoid unwanted pregnancy and sexually transmitted diseases and should be emphasized as the best choice for physical and emotional reasons.

Making a commitment to abstain from sexual activity

Practicing and using effective self-examination procedures

Chapter 3
Health Education

III. Expectations
and Content,
by Grade Level

Middle School

Unifying Idea:
Acceptance of personal
responsibility for
lifelong health

Expectation 2 (Continued)

Grade-level concepts and content	*Examples of skills and behaviors*

Treatment of disease:

Students at this level should be encouraged to take greater responsibility for the treatment of disease. They need to learn the symptoms of common diseases among youths and the importance of early diagnosis and treatment, including home treatment for common illnesses and the treatment and management of major diseases. In addition, they should learn when to seek qualified medical help. The curriculum should continue its focus on the importance of following prescribed health-care procedures and cooperating with parents and health-care providers to facilitate recovery or long-term treatment of diseases. Other topics appropriate for this grade span are the proper use of medication, including how to identify possible side effects, and personal rights and responsibilities involved in the treatment of disease. The influence of family and culture on the treatment of disease and the usefulness of participating in support groups or activities should continue to be explored.

■ Recognizing symptoms of common illnesses

■ Taking prescription and over-the-counter medicines properly

■ Interpreting correctly instructions written on medicine container labels, including using information provided with prescription and over-the-counter medicines to determine potential side effects

Determining when treatment of illness at home is appropriate and when and how to seek further help when needed

Accepting responsibility for active involvement in the treatment or management of disease, including practicing and using effective communication skills to discuss illness with parents and health-care providers

■ Identifies previously introduced skills or behaviors that should be built on and reinforced.

Expectation 3

Students will practice behaviors that reduce the risk of becoming involved in potentially dangerous situations and react to potentially dangerous situations in ways that help to protect their health.

Chapter 3
Health Education

III. Expectations
and Content,
by Grade Level

Middle School

Unifying Idea:
Acceptance of personal
responsibility for
lifelong health

Grade-level concepts and content	*Examples of skills and behaviors*

Potentially dangerous situations:

Because students in this age group may be especially prone to high-risk behavior, they should be given special instruction in ways to safeguard their lives. For example, they should be made familiar with the basic rules of traffic safety, including rules for drivers, occupants of motor vehicles, bicyclists, and pedestrians. And they should be taught to understand that traffic safety requires being observant at all times because others may not obey the rules.

Many potentially dangerous situations can be avoided or handled through the practice of safety precautions and the use of safety equipment in daily living. Students should learn to identify hazards found in the home, school, and community and participate in activities to remove those hazards.

Students should understand how to minimize the potential for injury when interacting with others who exhibit dangerous behavior. Violence threatens the safety of individuals and society. Effective instruction in violence prevention should include opportunities to practice nonharmful conflict-resolution strategies, including identification of the variety of factors that can influence such resolution. Students should

■ Developing and using appropriate skills to identify, avoid when possible, and cope with potentially dangerous situations, with emphasis on how peers can help each other avoid or cope with potentially dangerous situations in healthy ways

■ Practicing safe behavior in and near motorized vehicles

■ Practicing safe behavior in recreational activities, even in the absence of adults

■ Practicing safe behavior in and near water

■ Using appropriate skills to avoid, resolve, and cope with conflicts

■ Understanding and following rules prohibiting possession of weapons at school

■ Reporting or obtaining assistance when faced with unsafe situations

Identifying factors that reduce risks of accidents and demonstrating corrective action

Identifying environmental factors that affect health and safety

Recognizing that the use of alcohol and other drugs plays a role in many dangerous situations

■ Identifies previously introduced skills or behaviors that should be built on and reinforced.

Chapter 3
Health Education

III. Expectations
and Content,
by Grade Level

Middle School

Unifying Idea:
Acceptance of personal
responsibility for
lifelong health

Expectation 3 (Continued)

Grade-level concepts and content	*Examples of skills and behaviors*
Potentially dangerous situations:	
understand the importance of obeying school rules prohibiting the possession and use of weapons.	Demonstrating how peers can help each other avoid and cope with potentially dangerous situations in healthy ways Using thinking and decision-making skills in high-risk situations involving the use of motor vehicles and other hazardous activities
Alcohol, tobacco, and other drugs:	
The use of alcohol, tobacco, or other drugs frequently plays a role in the dangerous behaviors of adolescents and adults. Students should understand the short-term and long-term effects of using such substances, including those that may alter performance, such as steroids. Their effects on the health of unborn children should also be explored. Students should develop their understanding of the concept of chemical dependency and the effects of such dependency on the body. Another concern should be the effects on society of the use of alcohol, tobacco, and other drugs. Students should learn what laws (local, state, and federal), school policies, and family rules govern the use of chemical substances and should understand the consequences of illegal use of drugs. They should also be taught to understand the influence of peers and the media on the use of alcohol, tobacco, and other drugs; develop knowledge, skills, and strategies for choosing not to use or distribute such substances;	■ Exercising self-control ■ Developing and using interpersonal and other communication skills, such as assertiveness, refusal, negotiation, and conflict-resolution skills to avoid the use of alcohol, tobacco, and other drugs ■ Distinguishing between helpful and harmful substances ■ Differentiating between the use and misuse of prescription and nonprescription drugs ■ Avoiding, recognizing, and responding to negative social influences and pressure to use alcohol, tobacco, or other drugs ■ Using positive peer pressure to help counteract the negative effects of living in an environment where alcohol, tobacco, or other drug abuse or dependency exists ■ Identifying ways of obtaining help to resist pressure to use alcohol, tobacco, or other drugs

■ Identifies previously introduced skills or behaviors that should be built on and reinforced.

Chapter 3
Health Education

III. Expectations
and Content,
by Grade Level

Middle School

Unifying Idea:
Acceptance of personal
responsibility for
lifelong health

Grade-level concepts and content	*Examples of skills and behaviors*

Alcohol, tobacco, and other drugs:

and learn strategies for avoiding drug-related risk-taking situations and should have opportunities to practice those strategies. Numerous resources in the school and the community are available for people who have problems related to alcohol or drugs. However, many of the risk factors associated with the use of alcohol, tobacco, and other drugs are outside the student's control. A history of alcoholism at home, for example, or the easy availability of other drugs in the home or neighborhood are realities for many students. Even in adverse circumstances, however, students can learn and practice coping strategies that will reduce the risks. Students should know how and where to obtain help when confronted with alcohol- or drug-related problems.	Identifying and participating in positive alternative activities, such as alcohol-, tobacco-, and drug-free events

Child abuse, including sexual exploitation:

Information on the neglect and abuse of children should continue to be presented. Students should be told forcefully that these problems are serious and that they may require outside assistance. After parents are notified of the forthcoming instruction, students should also be provided with information on sexual abuse and rape. In addition, students should be helped to develop skills enabling them to prevent, avoid, and cope with unwanted sexual advances and be asked to demonstrate those skills. The skills include ability to assess	■ Identifying ways to seek assistance if concerned, abused, or threatened ■ Recognizing and avoiding situations that can increase risk of abuse Avoiding, recognizing, and responding to negative social influences and pressure to become sexually active, including applying refusal skills when appropriate

■ Identifies previously introduced skills or behaviors that should be built on and reinforced.

Chapter 3
Health Education

III. Expectations
and Content,
by Grade Level

Middle School

Unifying Idea:
Acceptance of personal
responsibility for
lifelong health

Expectation 3 (Continued)

Grade-level concepts and content	*Examples of skills and behaviors*

Child abuse, including sexual exploitation:

situations that may be dangerous; avoid those situations; avoid alcohol and other drug use; develop assertiveness skills; and learn self-defense techniques. Even when precautions are taken, however, sexual abuse or rape may occur. For that reason students should be made aware of and be given access to resources available for those who have been sexually abused, molested, or assaulted.

Emergencies:

Building on the knowledge and skills learned in the elementary grades, students should explore how to develop a detailed family emergency plan and maintain safety equipment and supplies in readiness for emergencies and natural disasters. Community emergency services should be analyzed, and effective means for using them should be explored. In addition to the first-aid skills learned in the upper elementary grades, students at this level should have the opportunity to demonstrate proficiency in standard first-aid procedures, abdominal-thrust maneuver, and cardiopulmonary resuscitation (CPR). Some students may have fears about contracting a disease while administering first aid or CPR. Because some of those fears are based on myth and some on fact, students should be provided with scientific data so that they can distinguish a genuine danger from a mistaken one.

■ Recognizing emergencies and responding appropriately, including demonstrating proficiency in basic first-aid procedures, abdominal thrust maneuver, and cardiopulmonary resuscitation (CPR)

Developing and maintaining, with other family members, a personal and family emergency plan, including maintaining supplies in readiness for emergencies

■ Identifies previously introduced skills or behaviors that should be built on and reinforced.

109

Chapter 3
Health Education

III. Expectations
and Content,
by Grade Level

Middle School

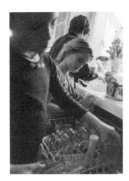

Unifying Idea
Respect for and promotion of the health of others

Expectations:

4. Students will understand and demonstrate how to play a positive, active role in promoting the health of their families.

5. Students will understand and demonstrate how to promote positive health practices within the school and community, including how to cultivate positive relationships with their peers.

Expectation 4

Students will understand and demonstrate how to play a positive, active role in promoting the health of their families.

Grade-level concepts and content	Examples of skills and behaviors
Roles of family members:	

Students should recognize that parenting can be a rich and rewarding experience but requires time and commitment. Parenting involves moral, social, legal, and financial responsibilities and is, therefore, an activity appropriate for responsible adults only. Parental responsibilities begin even prior to conception because health-related behavior of both parents before and during pregnancy influences the health of the baby. Although various cultures and societies have unique parenting patterns, all parents must provide for their children's development. As students explore the roles of parents, they should recognize that balancing the responsibilities of work and parenting can be difficult. Being a responsible parent means considering this challenge and striking an appropriate balance between work	▪ Supporting and valuing all family members ▪ Demonstrating ways in which children can help support positive family interactions ▪ Developing and using effective communication techniques, including talking openly and honestly with parents when problems arise and developing skills for discussing with parents questions about sexuality ▪ Practicing health-promoting behaviors with the family; recognizing its role in supporting positive health practices of others, especially younger children; and encouraging other family members to practice those positive behaviors Completing self-initiated activities beyond assigned chores to help

▪ Identifies previously introduced skills or behaviors that should be built on and reinforced.

Chapter 3
Health Education

III. Expectations
and Content,
by Grade Level

Middle School

Unifying Idea:
Respect for and
promotion of the
health of others

Expectation 4 (Continued)

Grade-level concepts and content	Examples of skills and behaviors
Roles of family members:	

and parenting. Students should also explore ways in which parental behavior affects children and focus on ways in which social, economic, and cultural factors affect family life. For example, the values or religious beliefs that parents teach and model influence how children behave. Students should recognize that traditions, history, and family pride are passed on by parents and extended family members.

One emphasis of the curriculum at this level should be on the difficulty and challenges of being a teenage parent. Teenagers are still growing and developing. Parenting responsibilities at that age can interrupt schooling, employment plans, and social and family life for both male and female teenagers. Further, the children of teenage parents often have more problems than do the children of adult parents. Birth defects, more common in children of teenage parents, are one example. In summary, teenage pregnancy can have serious effects on the teenage parent, the child, the teenager's family, and society.

Students should continue to identify the skills needed to be responsible family members and should have opportunities to practice those skills. They should recognize their role in promoting the health of family members as well as preventing injuries and promoting safety at home. As students explore their roles

support the family, such as doing the dishes without being asked

Identifying safety hazards in the home and helping to remove those hazards

Grade-level concepts and content	Examples of skills and behaviors

Roles of family members:

in their families, they should recognize that the responsibilities of children change as they grow older. With adolescence usually comes greater independence and often greater responsibility.

As the child's role in the family changes, good communication with parents is particularly important. Effective communication skills can be developed that can help adolescents and their parents talk about difficult subjects in a reasonable way. Students can also explore the effects emotions have on behaviors and communication. At times a cooling-off period may be needed before conflicts can be resolved. The importance of honesty, trust, and mutual respect in family communication should be emphasized. Occasional conflicts between parents and adolescents are normal. Positive ways to resolve conflict should be a continuing emphasis of the curriculum.

Change within the family:

Family interactions can be affected by changes in the family structure, including the results of unexpected change, disappointment, or grief. Yet there are healthy ways to deal with these emotions. Coping strategies can be developed, and family members can help each other through difficult times. Families sometimes need counseling to function well.

■ Using effective strategies to cope with change in the family, such as seeking assistance from a parent, a trusted adult, a support system, or counseling when needed

■ Identifies previously introduced skills or behaviors that should be built on and reinforced.

Chapter 3
Health Education

III. Expectations
and Content,
by Grade Level

Middle School

Unifying Idea:
Respect for and
promotion of the
health of others

Expectation 5

Students will understand and demonstrate how to promote positive health practices within the school and community, including how to cultivate positive relationships with their peers.

Grade-level concepts and content	*Examples of skills and behaviors*
Friendship and peer relationships:	

Positive peer relationships in adolescence are a key to good health. Students should be encouraged to reach out to and include others; conversely, they should be discouraged from becoming exclusive and clique-oriented. The curriculum should focus on the need to respect the dignity of all people, including students and adults at school, and to avoid name calling, prejudice, exclusiveness, discrimination, and conflict. Students should be reminded that, although they may not like everyone with whom they interact, it is important to be able to communicate and work effectively with a variety of people.

Students should demonstrate decision-making and problem-solving skills to enhance interpersonal relationships and skills for building and maintaining friendships. They should be encouraged to recognize the role of positive peer relationships in encouraging healthy behaviors and discouraging risk-taking behaviors. Emphasis on skills for influencing others to avoid the use of alcohol, tobacco, and other drugs as well as other unhealthy behaviors (such as eating disorders, unsafe behaviors in and

- ▨ Knowing and using appropriate ways to make new friends
- ▨ Demonstrating acceptable methods of gaining attention
- ▨ Demonstrating acceptable ways to show or express feelings
- ▨ Demonstrating positive actions toward others
- ▨ Resolving conflicts in a positive, constructive way
- ▨ Demonstrating how to resist negative peer pressure

Avoiding demeaning statements directed toward others

Interacting effectively with many different people, including both males and females and members of different ethnic and cultural groups

Promoting positive health behaviors among peers, including acknowledging and supporting the special health needs of others

Helping peers know when they should seek help from a parent or other trusted adult

▨ Identifies previously introduced skills or behaviors that should be built on and reinforced.

Chapter 3
Health Education

III. Expectations
and Content,
by Grade Level

Middle School

Unifying Idea:
Respect for and
promotion of the
health of others

Grade-level concepts and content	*Examples of skills and behaviors*

Friendship and peer relationships:

around motor vehicles, and unsafe risk-taking behaviors around bodies of water) should be continued at this level.

Because students at this level are likely to be interested in attending coeducational social activities, they should be encouraged to develop positive relationships with both males and females. Good communication is important in the development of positive relationships. Communication skills and the causes and consequences of miscommunication, should be explored.

School and community-based efforts to promote and protect health:

As students become more aware of and involved with the larger environment, they should have opportunities to examine how laws, policies, and practices influence health locally, nationally, and internationally. The curriculum should include descriptions of how public health efforts have helped to prevent, control, and eradicate disease and how personal and public actions have affected the environment. To be included is the role of public agencies in establishing rules and laws to protect community health now and in the future.

Students can also explore and participate in efforts by school and community organizations to improve health at local, national, and

- Understanding and following school rules related to health

- Participating in school efforts to promote health

- Assuming responsibility for helping to take care of the school, such as picking up trash on the school grounds and helping other students assume responsibility for that action

- Participating in community efforts to address local health and environmental issues

- Contributing to the strengthening of health-related policies at school

Encouraging others to become involved in health-promotion efforts at school

▪ Identifies previously introduced skills or behaviors that should be built on and reinforced.

Chapter 3
Health Education

III. Expectations
and Content,
by Grade Level

Middle School

Expectation 5 (Continued)

Grade-level concepts and content	*Examples of skills and behaviors*

School and community-based efforts to promote and protect health:

international levels. This is an appropriate time to introduce information about agencies and organizations that provide protection against fraudulent health products, services, and information. The curriculum can also include a study of food additives, recycling, food waste, hunger, pesticide use, and the need for a safe and adequate food supply. Students should promote activities centering on disease prevention among family and friends and learn ways to assist others in making positive health decisions that have an effect on themselves and others.	Analyzing the impact of laws, policies, and practices on health-related issues Encouraging others to become involved in health-promotion efforts at many different levels; for example choosing not to smoke, supporting the school as a tobacco-free environment, and supporting local efforts to reduce smoking in the community Accessing appropriately services available within the community

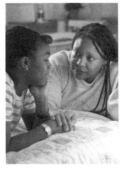

Unifying Idea
An understanding of the process of growth and development

Expectations:

6. Students will understand the variety of physical, mental, emotional, and social changes that occur throughout life.

7. Students will understand and accept individual differences in growth and development.

8. Students will understand their developing sexuality, will choose to abstain from sexual activity, will learn about protecting their sexual health, and will treat the sexuality of others with respect.

Expectation 6

Students will understand the variety of physical, mental, emotional, and social changes that occur throughout life.

Grade-level concepts and content	Examples of skills and behaviors
Life cycle:	

Middle School

Unifying Idea:
An understanding of
the process of growth
and development

Early adolescence and adolescence are times of intense change, growth, and development. They can also be times of emotional turmoil, uncertainty, anxiety, and related health and behavior problems. If not presented earlier, the changes associated with puberty and the structure and function of the male and female reproductive systems should be presented at this level. In addition to learning to understand the changes occurring during adolescence, students should be encouraged to develop strategies for coping with concerns and stress related to those changes.	■ Practicing good personal hygiene, paying particular attention to the changing needs of adolescents ■ Managing feelings appropriately ■ Developing and using effective communication skills to discuss with parents or other trusted adults the changes that occur during adolescence Recognizing fluctuations in emotions Practicing behaviors that will provide the option of healthy parenting later in life, such as avoidance of substance abuse

Expectation 7

Students will understand and accept individual differences in growth and development.

Growth and development:	

At a time when students are developing in different ways and at varying rates, differences in physical, mental, emotional, and social growth and development during adolescence are an appropriate focus of the curriculum. Students should understand that each person experiences change at his or her own pace. There is no exact time frame or	■ Demonstrating an understanding of individual differences ■ Adapting group activities to include a variety of students ■ Developing a realistic body image ■ Recognizing problems associated with not having a realistic body image, including dieting and

■ Identifies previously introduced skills or behaviors that should be built on and reinforced.

Chapter 3
Health Education

III. Expectations
and Content,
by Grade Level

Middle School

Unifying Idea:
An understanding of
the process of growth
and development

Expectation 7 (Continued)

Grade-level concepts and content	*Examples of skills and behaviors*

Growth and development:

age for particular changes to occur. In addition, students should understand the negative impact that alcohol, tobacco, and other drugs, including performance-altering substances, have on the body and develop strategies for avoiding the use of those substances.	eating disorders, and seeking appropriate help

Recognizing the effects of performance-altering substances and avoiding the use of those substances |

Mental and emotional development:

Although individuals vary greatly in their physical, mental, emotional, and social development, students should understand that all people face decisions that can influence future choices. Setting short-term and long-term goals is a helpful way of focusing and guiding one's life. While acknowledging the role of heredity in growth and development, students should be encouraged to set short-term and long-term goals related to personal health and physical fitness.	▪ Identifying, expressing, and managing feelings appropriately

▪ Developing and using effective communication skills

▪ Recognizing one's own strengths and limitations

▪ Using coping strategies, including time-management skills

Developing a focus on the future |

Expectation 8

Students will understand their developing sexuality, will choose to abstain from sexual activity, will learn about protecting their sexual health, and will treat the sexuality of others with respect.

Sexuality:

Note: The *Education Code* requires that parents be notified before any discussion of human reproductive organs and their functions and processes takes place.	Developing and using effective communication skills, including the ability to discuss with parents questions on sexuality

▪ Identifies previously introduced skills or behaviors that should be built on and reinforced.

Grade-level concepts and content	*Examples of skills and behaviors*

Sexuality:

Sexuality is a natural and healthy part of life. At this level it is appropriate to address the psychological, social, moral, and ethical aspects of sexuality. Students should recognize that there are differences and similarities between male and female sexuality and that the consequences of sexual involvement may differ. For example, teenage pregnancy usually has a greater impact on the female partner.

Abstinence from sexual activity should be an important theme in the curriculum at this level and should be emphasized as the wisest and healthiest choice for young people until marriage. Further, abstinence is the only totally effective method of contraception. All other methods of contraception carry a risk of failure in preventing unwanted teenage pregnancy. Statistics on the effectiveness or ineffectiveness of other birth-control methods in preventing unwanted pregnancies must be provided to students. Students who are considering sexual activity should be encouraged to talk with a parent or other trusted adult.

All students should be made aware that sexual feelings and desires are natural but should also be taught to recognize that they do not have to act on those feelings. They should be helped to understand that they can show affection in ways other than sexually and that love should not be equated with sexual involvement. Moreover, they must learn that it is

Identifying appropriate ways to show affection

Recognizing and avoiding situations that place one at risk of participating in sexual activity

Avoiding, recognizing, and responding to negative social influences and pressure to become sexually active

Demonstrating assertive and refusal skills and applying those skills to situations involving pressure to be sexually active

Identifying ways to seek assistance if abused

Practicing behaviors that support the decision to abstain from sexual activity

III. Expectations
and Content,
by Grade Level

Middle School

Unifying Idea:
An understanding of
the process of growth
and development

Middle School

Unifying Idea:
An understanding of
the process of growth
and development

Expectation 8 (Continued)

Grade-level concepts and content	*Examples of skills and behaviors*
Sexuality:	

never appropriate to force someone to have any type of intimate sexual contact.

A factual, substantiated discussion of homosexuality may be presented at this level. (*Note:* School district governing boards considering approval of such a discussion should refer to "Family Living" in Section II of this chapter and to Appendix A.) The discussion might be conducted in a limited way during or after grade seven and more fully in high school. Students should recognize, however, that most persons feel affection for both men and women and that affection for someone of the same sex is not necessarily an indicator of homosexuality. Teenagers questioning their sexual orientation may be reluctant to discuss the topic for fear of reprisal. Students should respect the rights of others to seek information about homosexuality from a parent or other trusted and knowledgeable adult.

The California Student Safety and Violence Prevention Act of 2000 (AB 537) promotes an appreciation of diversity in a democratic society. Name-calling or other hurtful actions must not be tolerated. Teachers, counselors, physicians, religious leaders, and community resource centers may offer support for young people who have concerns about their sexual orientation. Religious and personal beliefs should be respected, and instruction should affirm the dignity of all people.

119

Chapter 3
Health Education

III. Expectations
and Content,
by Grade Level

Middle School

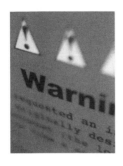

Unifying Idea

Informed use of health-related information, products, and services

Expectation:

9. Students will identify information, products, and services that may be helpful or harmful to their health.

Expectation 9

Students will identify information, products, and services that may be helpful or harmful to their health.

Grade-level concepts and content	Examples of skills and behaviors

Products and services:

At this level students should be encouraged to analyze in depth the range of health services in the community available from public and private organizations and agencies. They should identify those services that seek to prevent and treat disease. At the same time students should be encouraged to distinguish health concerns they can manage from those that require professional care. The relationship of values, socioeconomic status, and cultural experiences to the selection of health-care services should be emphasized.

Health fads and misconceptions about treatment and prevention options are appropriate for exploration, including the influence of advertising on the selection of health products and services. Students should have opportunities to contrast advertised images with real images. For example, they might

- Identifying a variety of consumer influences and analyzing how those influences affect decisions

- Recognizing helpful products and services

- Using critical-thinking skills to analyze marketing and advertising techniques and their influence on the selection of health-related services and products

- Seeking care from the school nurse or school-linked services with families when appropriate

Identifying appropriate sources of health services for a variety of illnesses

Developing and applying criteria for the selection or rejection of health products, services, and information, such as determining when appropriate to take a vitamin or mineral supplement

■ Identifies previously introduced skills or behaviors that should be built on and reinforced.

Chapter 3
Health Education

III. Expectations
and Content,
by Grade Level

Middle School

Unifying Idea:
Informed use of
health-related
information,
products,
and services

Expectation 9 (Continued)

Grade-level concepts and content	*Examples of skills and behaviors*

Products and services:

counter the advertised image of youth and rugged good health or a happy cartoon character in tobacco ads with diseases caused by smoking that ravage a smoker's health.

Students should develop criteria for the selection or rejection of health products, services, and information. They should be able to analyze labels on health-related products to determine whether the products are appropriate for personal use and when they might be used. The qualifications of various health-care providers should be explored. Because the opinions of health-care professionals are not infallible, there may be legitimate reasons for requesting additional information or a second opinion. Students should be able to recognize when they might wish to obtain additional information or a second opinion and analyze how to obtain this information or service. The curriculum should also include an exploration of health- and food-related careers.

Food choices:

Increasingly, students at this grade span purchase or prepare their own meals and snacks at home or away from home. They need to be aware of the variety of low-cost foods that provide nutritionally adequate diets. Information should also be provided on reliable sources

- Using labels to compare the contents of food products

- Using critical-thinking skills to analyze marketing and advertising techniques and their influence on food selection

▨ Identifies previously introduced skills or behaviors that should be built on and reinforced.

121

Chapter 3
Health Education

III. Expectations
and Content,
by Grade Level

Middle School

Unifying Idea:
Informed use of
health-related
information,
products,
and services

Grade-level concepts and content	Examples of skills and behaviors

Food choices:

of nutrition information. Students need to develop skills in identifying and responding to influences—from peers, family, friends, the media, advertising, and industry—that influence personal food choices.

■ Using valid nutrition information to make healthy food choices

■ Using unit pricing to determine the most economical purchases

■ Developing basic food-preparation skills, including safe and sanitary food preparation and storage

Because eating disorders and fad dieting can lead to serious health problems, students should guard against becoming victims of media and peer pressures that promote an idealized and unattainable body image inappropriate for most persons. Adolescents need to be especially wary of nutrition and health claims that promise unrealistic results.

Using effective consumer skills to purchase healthy foods within budget constraints in a variety of settings

Using critical-thinking skills to distinguish facts from fallacies concerning the nutritional value of foods and food supplements

Adapting recipes to make them more healthy by lowering fat, salt, or sugar and increasing fiber

Using critical-thinking skills to analyze weight modification practices and selecting appropriate practices to maintain, lose, or gain weight according to individual need and scientific research

■ Identifies previously introduced skills or behaviors that should be built on and reinforced.

122

Chapter 3
Health Education

III. Expectations
and Content,
by Grade Level

High School

Several principles should be kept in mind when developing health education for students in high school. First, although many students may seem physically mature, they are still in the process of changing from external guidance to internal direction. In addition, the illusion of immortality is common to them, and the possibility of their developing a disease or disability in the distant future may carry even less weight for them than for younger adolescents. Therefore, instruction centering on the more immediate consequences of behavior or the imminent transition to adulthood is likely to be more effective than instruction emphasizing a long-term approach. Students are receptive to information provided by trusted adults but are often overconfident about their own knowledge and coping abilities. Therefore, positive adult and peer role models are critically important at this stage.

A positive development among many students is that they are becoming aware of their influence on younger children and are taking an increasingly active role in the school and the community as concerned citizens. They are often willing participants as role models or peer advisers. By this time most students are also beginning to think about career and life options. The curriculum can stimulate those interests and help to inform students about health- or food-related careers.

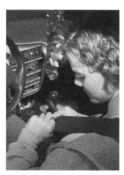

Unifying Idea
Acceptance of personal responsibility for lifelong health

Expectations:

1. Students will demonstrate ways in which they can enhance and maintain their health and well-being.
2. Students will understand and demonstrate behaviors that prevent disease and speed recovery from illness.
3. Students will practice behaviors that reduce the risk of becoming involved in potentially dangerous situations and react to potentially dangerous situations in ways that help to protect their health.

Chapter 3
Health Education

III. Expectations
and Content,
by Grade Level

High School

Unifying Idea:
Acceptance of personal
responsibility for
lifelong health

Expectation 1

Students will demonstrate ways in which they can enhance and maintain their health and well-being.

Grade-level concepts and content	*Examples of skills and behaviors*
The human body:	

The relationship among personal health habits, personal health, and the quality of life continues to be an important focus at this grade level. Students should develop a plan of health habits appropriate to their individual needs and analyze the ways in which personal health needs change during the life cycle. In addition, students should analyze how environmental conditions affect body systems and be able to demonstrate ways to protect themselves from exposure to potentially harmful conditions.

■ Practicing good personal hygiene

■ Using protective equipment, such as a helmet when cycling, or practicing behaviors to protect the body, such as avoiding exposure to excessive noises

■ Recognizing and accepting differences in body types and maturation levels

Responding appropriately to the physical development of older adolescents in ways that promote physical health through such preventive measures as healthy food choices and exercise

Food choices:	

The curriculum should emphasize nutritional needs during the different life stages—for example, prenatal development, infancy, early childhood, adolescence, and adulthood. Individual dietary requirements vary by age, gender, health status, and level of activity. The unique nutritional needs of adolescents, including pregnant teenagers and school-age parents, should be particularly emphasized.

The effects of nutrition and exercise on behavior, appearance, and physical and mental performance

■ Making healthy food choices in a variety of settings

■ Establishing and maintaining healthy eating practices, including developing and using a personal nutrition plan based on food choices and calorie levels that promotes health and reduces risk of disease

■ Analyzing how food choices are influenced, including how a busy schedule influences food choices

■ Selecting appropriate practices to maintain, lose, or gain weight

■ Identifies previously introduced skills or behaviors that should be built on and reinforced.

Chapter 3
Health Education

III. Expectations
and Content,
by Grade Level

High School

Unifying Idea:
Acceptance of personal
responsibility for
lifelong health

Expectation 1 (Continued)

Grade-level concepts and content	*Examples of skills and behaviors*

Food choices:

should also be highlighted, together with the role of nutrition in preventing chronic disease. Students should develop a culturally appropriate, long-range personal nutrition plan, based on food choices and calorie levels, that promotes health and reduces the risk of disease. They should be aware of the various food sources of nutrients available in different cultural and ethnic cuisines. They should also practice healthy food-preparation skills at home, at school, and in the community.

based on individual needs and scientific research

Recognizing the need for updating the personal nutrition plan as individual needs or activities change and being able to do so

Physical activity:

The curriculum should continue to emphasize the pleasure of physical activity. Students should be encouraged to explore a variety of activities in school and outside school. They should explore the connections between physical activity and mental and emotional health. As students plan for their transition to adulthood, they should investigate ways to maintain regular exercise practices and explore the potential harm of a sedentary lifestyle.

A periodic self-assessment of physical fitness should be a regular practice for students at this level. Assessment results should be used to evaluate progress toward meeting personal physical fitness goals and to refine personal fitness programs as necessary. Students should also

■ Observing safety rules during physical activities

■ Exploring ways to engage in out-of-school activities that promote health

■ Participating regularly in a variety of enjoyable physical activities

■ Following through with a personal fitness plan based on personal fitness goals and the results of periodic self-assessments

Making the adjustments needed for successful implementation of the personal fitness plan, including getting additional rest when necessary

■ Identifies previously introduced skills or behaviors that should be built on and reinforced.

Chapter 3
Health Education

III. Expectations
and Content,
by Grade Level

High School

Unifying Idea:
Acceptance of personal
responsibility for
lifelong health

Grade-level concepts and content	Examples of skills and behaviors

Physical activity:

discuss and analyze factors that influence personal motivation for participating in regular physical activity. If appropriate, they should be encouraged to develop self-motivation and self-discipline strategies to achieve personal goals. Students should be encouraged to accept differences among individuals and recognize that different activities appeal to different people.	Analyzing personal motivators related to pursuing physical activity and using those motivators to maintain ongoing participation in physical activities

Exploring ways to continue regular exercise practices when schedules change, such as during travel or while working |

Mental and emotional health:

The mental and emotional aspects of health continue to be strongly emphasized in the curriculum at this level. Students should have opportunities to recognize and build on personal characteristics that contribute to self-confidence and self-esteem. They should understand that usually there is more than one way to solve a problem and should have opportunities to practice problem-solving skills. Students should continue to be encouraged to pursue leisure-time activities that promote physical and mental health.

The topic of suicide, introduced in middle school, can be explored in more depth at this level. Students who feel rejected or socially isolated should be encouraged to develop strategies for coping with and overcoming these feelings. Acceptable alternatives include talking over problems, understanding that feelings of depression and isolation | ▪ Demonstrating personal characteristics that contribute to self-confidence and self-esteem, such as honesty, integrity, responsibility, and respect for the dignity of others

▪ Developing protective factors that help promote resiliency, such as developing an internal focus of control and maintaining a future focus

▪ Developing and using effective communication skills

▪ Developing and using effective coping strategies

▪ Avoiding self-destructive behaviors

▪ Practicing strategies for resisting negative peer pressure

▪ Identifying the strongest risk factors for negative behaviors in their own lives and developing effective strategies for counteracting the effect of those risk factors |

▪ Identifies previously introduced skills or behaviors that should be built on and reinforced.

III. Expectations
and Content,
by Grade Level

High School

Unifying Idea:
Acceptance of personal
responsibility for
lifelong health

Expectation 1 (Continued)

Grade-level concepts and content	*Examples of skills and behaviors*

Mental and emotional health:

will pass, examining the situation leading to the problem, seeking appropriate assistance if depression persists, obtaining medical treatment for organically caused depression, and participating in regular aerobic exercise. Students should understand the role of denial as a negative influence on mental and emotional health and should have opportunities to develop and use effective communication skills to overcome denial and seek assistance when needed.

- Selecting entertainment that promotes mental and physical health

Identifying personal habits influencing mental and emotional health and developing strategies for changing behaviors as needed to promote positive mental and emotional health

Relating in positive ways to peers and adults in and out of school

Expectation 2

Students will understand and demonstrate behaviors that prevent disease and speed recovery from illness.

Disease prevention:

At this level students should receive more detailed information on communicable and chronic diseases and disorders. In addition, future trends and the social and economic impact of such diseases and disorders on people and society should be discussed. Students should learn about the major communicable and chronic diseases prevalent at different stages of life and be able to explain how the immune system functions to prevent or combat disease. A variety of ways to prevent the major diseases should be described. The importance of prenatal and perinatal care and the impact of

- Practicing good personal hygiene to prevent the spread of disease
- Practicing positive health behaviors to reduce the risk of disease
- Cooperating in regular health screenings, including dental examinations
- Demonstrating safe care and concern toward ill persons in the family, school, and community
- Making a commitment to abstain from sexual activity, including exploring nonphysical ways to express affection
- Practicing and using effective self-examination procedures

- Identifies previously introduced skills or behaviors that should be built on and reinforced.

Chapter 3
Health Education

III. Expectations
and Content,
by Grade Level

High School

Unifying Idea:
Acceptance of personal
responsibility for
lifelong health

Grade-level concepts and content	*Examples of skills and behaviors*

Disease prevention:

this care on both the woman and her child should also be stressed. This framework encourages emphasis on both prenatal and perinatal care so that students will understand the benefits of prenatal care to the woman and her child and the importance of care after delivery, especially for the newborn. Students should be encouraged to practice specific behaviors that support those who are ill but avoid contagion.

Continued emphasis should be given to the prevention of sexually transmitted diseases, especially HIV/AIDS. Students should compare the effectiveness of abstinence with the effectiveness or ineffectiveness of other methods of preventing sexually transmitted diseases.

The importance of regular examinations, including self-examination of the breasts or testicles, in detecting and treating diseases early should be emphasized at this time. Students should learn how to discuss procedures and test results with their health-care providers.

Recognizing the importance of prenatal and perinatal care

Analyzing personal behaviors to determine how those behaviors relate to their own health and well-being and the fulfillment of personal goals and how those behaviors can be modified if necessary to promote achievement of those goals

Treatment of disease:

Students should be encouraged to learn ways to become fully informed about personal illness, including how to analyze the symptoms of disease and how to communicate about one's personal health with health-care providers. Family, social, economic, and cultural influences also play a role

■ Recognizing symptoms of common illnesses

■ Taking prescription and over-the-counter medicines properly

■ Interpreting correctly the instructions written on medicine labels

■ Determining when treatment of illness at home is appropriate and

■ Identifies previously introduced skills or behaviors that should be built on and reinforced.

Chapter 3
Health Education

III. Expectations
and Content,
by Grade Level

High School

Unifying Idea:
Acceptance of personal
responsibility for
lifelong health

Expectation 2 (Continued)

Grade-level concepts and content	*Examples of skills and behaviors*

Treatment of disease:

in how people care for personal illness. The importance of cooperating with parents and health-care providers in the treatment or management of disease should be continually emphasized. Students should also analyze the beneficial effects of medications generally and explain why it is important to take or administer prescription and over-the-counter medicines responsibly. The influence of family and cultural factors on the treatment of disease and the usefulness of participating in support groups or activities should continue to be explored.	when and how to seek further help when needed

■ Accepting responsibility for active involvement in the treatment or management of disease, including practicing and using effective communication skills to discuss illness, test results, or procedures with parents and health-care providers

Interpreting correctly the information provided by health-care providers regarding test results or procedures

Analyzing one's patterns related to treatment of disease to determine whether those patterns are effective and changing behaviors if necessary to facilitate management or recovery |

Expectation 3

Students will practice behaviors that reduce the risk of becoming involved in potentially dangerous situations and react to potentially dangerous situations in ways that help to protect their health.

Grade-level concepts and content	*Examples of skills and behaviors*

Potentially dangerous situations:

Because many students begin driving automobiles during this period and because young drivers are at particularly high risk of being involved in automobile accidents, they should be taught the basic rules of traffic safety as an important focus	■ Developing and using appropriate skills to identify, avoid when possible, or cope with potentially dangerous situations

■ Practicing safe behavior in and near motorized vehicles, including observing basic traffic safety rules |

■ Identifies previously introduced skills or behaviors that should be built on and reinforced.

Chapter 3
Health Education

III. Expectations
and Content,
by Grade Level

High School

Unifying Idea:
Acceptance of personal
responsibility for
lifelong health

Grade-level concepts and content	Examples of skills and behaviors

Potentially dangerous situations:

of the curriculum. Students should understand that safety requires being observant at all times because others may not follow the rules of safe driving.

Many potentially dangerous situations can be avoided or handled by the observance of safety precautions and the use of safety equipment in everyday life. Students should learn to identify hazards found in the home, the school, and the community and participate in activities to remove those hazards. They should also have the opportunity to examine what constitutes a safe versus an unsafe neighborhood and be encouraged to participate in activities that promote neighborhood safety.

A firearm is a noteworthy example of a hazardous object. Students should learn that under no circumstances should they possess or touch a firearm except under the direction of a responsible adult. Students who will be handling firearms for recreation should take a firearm-safety training course.

Students should understand how to minimize the potential for injury when interacting with others who exhibit dangerous behavior. As in grades six through nine, students should be given opportunities to practice nonharmful conflict-resolution strategies and identify factors that can influence conflict resolution.

when driving, developing proficiency in handling a vehicle in difficult situations, wearing a seat belt, and ensuring that others wear seat belts

■ Practicing safe behavior in recreational activities, even in the absence of adults

■ Practicing safe behavior in and near water

■ Using appropriate skills to avoid, resolve, and cope with conflicts

■ Understanding and following rules prohibiting possession of weapons at school

■ Reporting or obtaining assistance when faced with unsafe situations

■ Identifying factors that reduce risks of accidents and demonstrating corrective action

■ Identifying environmental factors that affect health and safety

■ Recognizing that the use of alcohol, tobacco, and other drugs plays a role in many dangerous situations

■ Demonstrating how peers can help each other avoid or cope with potentially dangerous situations in healthy ways

■ Using thinking and decision-making skills in high-risk situations involving motor vehicles and other safety hazards

Carrying emergency equipment in their vehicle

Using latex gloves when assisting persons who are injured

■ Identifies previously introduced skills or behaviors that should be built on and reinforced.

Chapter 3
Health Education

III. Expectations
and Content,
by Grade Level

High School

Unifying Idea:
Acceptance of personal
responsibility for
lifelong health

Expectation 3 (Continued)

Grade-level concepts and content	*Examples of skills and behaviors*

Alcohol, tobacco, and other drugs:

The short-term and long-term effects associated with the use of alcohol, tobacco, and other drugs (including those that may alter performance, such as steroids), alone or in combination, including their effects on reproduction, pregnancy, and the health of children, should be emphasized at this level. Students should continue to explore the legal, social, and economic consequences of drug use. Instruction should continue to emphasize laws, school policies, and family rules governing the use of chemical substances. Students should also continue to develop knowledge, skills, and strategies for choosing not to use or distribute alcohol, tobacco, and other drugs. Included should be practice in ways to avoid situations involving alcohol, tobacco, and other drugs that can have a negative influence on the students' health.

Students should recognize that abuse of alcohol, tobacco, and other drugs frequently plays a role in dangerous behavior. Results of such behavior include house fires, motor-vehicle crashes, domestic violence, date rape, and the transmission of HIV/AIDS through needle sharing or sexual activity. Students should examine the influence of chemical use on driving ability, other physical tasks, and judgment and should have opportunities to practice both refusal skills and healthy responses to high-risk situations.

- Exercising self-control

- Developing and using interpersonal and other communication skills, such as assertiveness, refusal, negotiation, and conflict-resolution skills to avoid use of alcohol, tobacco, and other drugs

- Distinguishing between helpful and harmful substances

- Distinguishing between the use and misuse of prescription and nonprescription drugs

- Avoiding, recognizing, and responding to negative social influences and pressure to use alcohol, tobacco, or other drugs

- Using positive peer pressure to help counteract the negative effects of living in an environment in which abuse of or dependence on alcohol, tobacco, or other drugs is present

- Identifying ways to obtain help to resist pressures to use alcohol, tobacco, or other drugs

- Identifying and participating in positive alternatives, such as alcohol-, tobacco-, and drug-free events

Helping to develop and support the school's no-use policy and working to support it by knowing the procedures for reporting offenses and setting a positive example

■ Identifies previously introduced skills or behaviors that should be built on and reinforced.

Chapter 3
Health Education

III. Expectations
and Content,
by Grade Level

High School

Unifying Idea:
Acceptance of personal
responsibility for
lifelong health

Grade-level concepts and content	*Examples of skills and behaviors*

Alcohol, tobacco, and other drugs:

Information should be provided about resources in the school and community that can help people who have alcohol-, tobacco-, or drug-related problems. The curriculum should also explore the disease concept of chemical dependencies. Students should build on their understanding of the concept that although many of the risk factors associated with alcohol and other drug use are not under the student's control, students can learn and practice coping strategies that will diminish the risks. They should analyze the role of positive coping strategies and self-respect in counteracting peer and environmental pressure to use drugs.

Child abuse, including sexual exploitation:

Neglect and child abuse should continue to be considered. Emphasis should be placed on the fact that these are serious problems that may require outside assistance. After parents are notified, students should be given information on sexual abuse and rape. Skills related to preventing, avoiding, and coping with unwanted sexual advances can be developed, and students should demonstrate those skills. Even when precautions are taken, however, a rape may occur. Students should be aware of and be able to obtain help provided for those who have been sexually abused, molested, or assaulted.

- Identifying ways to seek assistance if concerned, abused, or threatened

- Recognizing and avoiding situations that can increase risk of abuse, including avoiding the use of alcohol and other drugs

- Avoiding, recognizing, and responding to negative social influences and pressure to become sexually active, including applying refusal skills when appropriate

- Developing and using assertiveness skills and learning self-defense techniques

■ Identifies previously introduced skills or behaviors that should be built on and reinforced.

High School

Unifying Idea:
Acceptance of personal
responsibility for
lifelong health

Expectation 3 (Continued)

Grade-level concepts and content	*Examples of skills and behaviors*
Emergencies:	

If not learned earlier, cardiopulmonary resuscitation (CPR) and other first-aid procedures for life-threatening emergencies should be mastered at this level. In addition to the skills listed at previous grade levels, instruction should include caring for victims of severe insect stings and snakebites as well as learning how to administer first aid to persons with broken bones and how to transport victims properly. The personal and legal responsibilities of persons involved in emergencies should be explored and analyzed. Students should continue to work with their families to identify and remove safety hazards in the home, develop and maintain a detailed family emergency plan, and maintain safety equipment and supplies for emergencies and natural disasters. Emergency supplies should be maintained at home and in vehicles. Students and their families should discuss what they would do if one or more family members were away from home during an emergency and include plans for coping with this situation in their family emergency plan. They should analyze local emergency services and determine the appropriate (and inappropriate) use of those services.	■ Recognizing emergency situations and responding appropriately ■ Developing and maintaining, with other family members, a personal and family emergency plan, including maintaining supplies in readiness for emergencies, including supplies at home and supplies in their vehicle Identifying appropriate use of local emergency services Using latex gloves when assisting persons who are injured

■ Identifies previously introduced skills or behaviors that should be built on and reinforced.

Chapter 3
Health Education

III. Expectations
and Content,
by Grade Level

High School

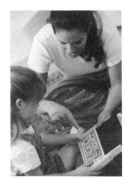

Unifying Idea
Respect for and promotion of the health of others

Expectations:

4. Students will understand and demonstrate how to play a positive, active role in promoting the health of their families.

5. Students will understand and demonstrate how to promote positive health practices within the school and community, including how to cultivate positive relationships with their peers.

Expectation 4

Students will understand and demonstrate how to play a positive, active role in promoting the health of their families.

Grade-level concepts and content	Examples of skills and behaviors
Roles of family members:	

Building on the information presented at earlier levels, students at this level should continue to explore family development and the factors that help families to stay strong and healthy, including the sharing of a variety of family experiences and traditions. Family communication remains an important area to emphasize, especially in light of the growing independence of adolescents.

Strong families help their members reach their fullest potential. Ways of strengthening families include continually emphasizing, within the family, ways to support and respect all family members, effective approaches for solving family problems, and strategies for dealing with crisis and change. As adolescents develop more independence from their parents, they may exhibit or be tempted to exhibit

▪ Supporting and valuing all family members

▪ Demonstrating ways in which adolescents can help support positive family interactions

▪ Developing and using effective communication techniques

▪ Practicing health-promoting behaviors with the family; recognizing their role in supporting positive health practices of others, especially younger children; and encouraging other family members to practice those positive behaviors

▪ Completing self-initiated activities beyond assigned chores to help support the family

▪ Identifying safety hazards in the home and helping to remove them

Seeking assistance if living in a family where abuse of alcohol or

▪ Identifies previously introduced skills or behaviors that should be built on and reinforced.

Chapter 3
Health Education

III. Expectations
and Content,
by Grade Level

High School

Unifying Idea:
Respect for and
promotion of the
health of others

Expectation 4 (Continued)

Grade-level concepts and content	*Examples of skills and behaviors*
### Roles of family members:	
individual behavior that conflicts with their family's standards. Students should understand how this behavior can affect the family and practice family communication skills and related approaches to solving family problems and conflicts. Instruction at this level should emphasize that family members can have conflicts while continuing to love and support each other. Students should analyze short-term and long-term effects that the abuse of alcohol, tobacco, or other drugs can have on the roles and relationships within the family. For example, some students at this age may take on roles inappropriate for their age but necessary because of family structure. For example, the oldest child of alcoholic parents may assume responsibility for monitoring and disciplining younger siblings.	other drugs exists (e.g., participating in support groups for teens who are the children of alcoholics)
### Change within the family:	
The effects of change on family interactions continue to be important at this grade span. The curriculum may include the influence of religious or cultural beliefs on family interactions. For example, students might analyze the process of grieving in various cultures. In addition, they should investigate their upcoming transition to independent living, critique their skills related to this transition, and create a plan to help develop those skills necessary for a	■ Using effective strategies to cope with change in the family Developing a plan to facilitate transition from the role as a child to the role of an independent adult and discussing the plan with one's parents while it is being developed Discussing with parents plans to continue education beyond high school and developing a mutual understanding of how this change will affect family roles and interactions

■ Identifies previously introduced skills or behaviors that should be built on and reinforced.

135

Chapter 3
Health Education

III. Expectations
and Content,
by Grade Level

High School

Unifying Idea:
Respect for and
promotion of the
health of others

Change within the family:

successful transition. Students should also explore how the aging process affects families and should understand their role in helping their parents assist grandparents.

Expectation 5

Students will understand and demonstrate how to promote positive health practices within the school and community, including how to cultivate positive relationships with their peers.

Grade-level concepts and content	*Examples of skills and behaviors*

Friendship and peer relationships:

An important emphasis of the curriculum at this level is the need to respect the dignity of all people. Students should demonstrate ability to interact effectively with a wide range of people at school and should encourage others to behave in similar positive ways toward others. It will be important to distinguish between one's own feelings about the opinions or behaviors of other people and the need to respect others' rights and individuality. That is, students should realize that one can disagree with others and still interact effectively with them.

Students should understand the importance of their personal standards being consistent with their behavior. They should demonstrate decision-making and problem-solving skills to enhance interpersonal relationships as well as skills for building and maintaining friendships. Positive, healthy

◼ Knowing and using appropriate ways to make new friends

◼ Demonstrating positive actions toward others

◼ Resolving conflicts in a positive, constructive way

◼ Demonstrating how to resist negative peer pressure

◼ Interacting effectively with many different people, including both males and females and members of different ethnic and cultural groups

◼ Avoiding demeaning statements directed toward others

◼ Promoting positive health behaviors among peers

Participating in group activities as a means of getting to know other people

Analyzing appropriate behaviors in a dating relationship

◼ Identifies previously introduced skills or behaviors that should be built on and reinforced.

Chapter 3
Health Education

III. Expectations
and Content,
by Grade Level

High School

Unifying Idea:
Respect for and
promotion of the
health of others

Expectation 5 (Continued)

Grade-level concepts and content	*Examples of skills and behaviors*

Friendship and peer relationships:

friendships reinforce one's sense of self-worth. Students should recognize the role of responsible companions in encouraging healthy behavior and discouraging unhealthy risk-taking, including strategies for influencing others to avoid the use of alcohol, tobacco, and other drugs as well as other negative behaviors.

Developing new friendships and new social skills with males and females should also be emphasized. Students should continue to develop and enhance their communication skills and skills for building and maintaining friendships. Group activities should be encouraged that allow teenagers to learn about others without dating. Students should recognize that people date for different reasons, that not all teenagers date, and that parents usually decide at what age their children may start dating. As they develop friendships, students can begin to identify criteria that might be used later in life to select a mate.

Honor and respect for monogamous, heterosexual marriage should be an important emphasis of the curriculum at this level. Students should be able to contrast a dating relationship with a marriage relationship. Dating can be a way to learn about other people, about romantic feelings and expressions, and about what it is like to be in a love relationship. Marriage is a legal commitment that a man and a woman make to

Respecting the dignity of the persons with whom they interact, including dates, and expecting that their own dignity will be treated with respect

Respecting monogamous, heterosexual marriage

137

Chapter 3
Health Education

III. Expectations
and Content,
by Grade Level

High School

Unifying Idea:
Respect for and
promotion of the
health of others

Grade-level concepts and content	*Examples of skills and behaviors*

Friendship and peer relationships:

share their lives and family responsibilities. It requires dedication and perseverance. A successful marriage requires good interpersonal skills and the ability to make adjustments to meet the needs of another person. The importance of open communication, respect, honesty, and monogamy in marriage should be emphasized.

School and community-based efforts to promote and protect health:

Building on their earlier study, students should evaluate local, national, and international efforts for preventing, controlling, and eradicating disease, hunger, and pollution. They should have opportunities to analyze how public health policies and laws are developed and to examine the role of interest groups and individual advocacy in this process and the importance of voting. Students should examine how nations share responsibility for the health of all people; for example, international response to disasters can be explored. In addition, they may initiate or participate in developing school and community efforts to prevent and control disease. Community responsibility for health promotion can also be explored through an analysis of the efforts of local government and community groups and organizations.

- Understanding and following school rules related to health

- Participating in school efforts to promote health

- Assuming responsibility for helping to take care of the school and helping other students assume responsibility for that task

- Participating in community efforts to address local health and environmental issues, such as volunteer work at hospitals, food banks, child-care centers, centers for persons recovering from trauma, or centers for persons with disabilities

- Encouraging others to become involved in health-promotion efforts at school

- Analyzing the influence of laws, policies, and practices on health-related issues, including those related to food and nutrition

■ Identifies previously introduced skills or behaviors that should be built on and reinforced.

High School

Unifying Idea:
Respect for and
promotion of the
health of others

Expectation 5 (Continued)

Grade-level concepts and content	*Examples of skills and behaviors*

School and community-based efforts to promote and protect health:

Students should also identify the psychosocial needs of those who are disabled or ill and analyze the services provided by community organizations and agencies in meeting these needs. For example, students might explore the services available to support patients afflicted by Alzheimer's disease and their families. Specific strategies for involving others in safely demonstrating care and concern for people who are ill should be included. Students should recognize that while anyone can become disabled, disabilities are not contagious.

Students can also analyze laws and standards related to food, food handling, an adequate food supply, the environment, and agriculture. They can become active in environmental and economic issues that affect the food supply and the nutritional quality of food.

- Encouraging others to become involved in health-promotion efforts at many different levels
- Accessing appropriately those services available within the community

Initiating and involving others in health-promotion efforts at school or in the community

■ Identifies previously introduced skills or behaviors that should be built on and reinforced.

139

Chapter 3
Health Education

III. Expectations
and Content,
by Grade Level

High School

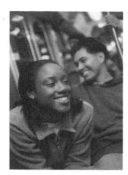

Unifying Idea
An understanding of the process of growth and development

Expectations:

6. Students will understand the variety of physical, mental, emotional, and social changes that occur throughout life.

7. Students will understand and accept individual differences in growth and development.

8. Students will understand their developing sexuality, will choose to abstain from sexual activity, will learn about protecting their sexual health, and will treat the sexuality of others with respect.

Expectation 6

Students will understand the variety of physical, mental, emotional, and social changes that occur throughout life

Grade-level concepts and content	*Examples of skills and behaviors*
Life cycle:	

The various stages of life, including pregnancy, infancy, childhood, adolescence, young adulthood, middle age, and older adulthood, should be investigated by students at this time. Students should recognize that a variety of physical, mental, emotional, and social changes occur throughout life and that although there are predictable stages of a human being's life cycle, people develop and mature at their own rate. A person's ability to make adjustments while passing through the various stages of life can significantly influence the quality of that life. Students should explore changes during the life cycle, including	■ Developing and using effective communication skills to discuss with parents or other trusted adults the changes that occur during adolescence ■ Practicing behaviors that will provide for healthy parenting later in life, such as avoidance of substance abuse Recognizing and being prepared to adapt to the changes that occur during life, such as changes associated with young adulthood, pregnancy, middle age, or old age Recognizing and acknowledging that different people progress through different stages of the life cycle at different rates

■ Identifies previously introduced skills or behaviors that should be built on and reinforced.

Chapter 3
Health Education

III. Expectations
and Content,
by Grade Level

High School

Unifying Idea:
An understanding of
the process of growth
and development

Expectation 6 (Continued)

Grade-level concepts and content	*Examples of skills and behaviors*

Life cycle:

normal bodily growth and development, and physical changes caused by diseases and injuries. They should investigate the influence of food choices on the various stages of life and on recovery from diseases and injuries. Students should also analyze how such skills as the ability to cope, adjust, make decisions, communicate feelings, make and keep friends, care for others, and show concern for the community influence individuals through the various stages of life.

This level is appropriate for emphasizing the reproductive process and fetal development from conception through pregnancy to birth. The curriculum should address the role of prenatal care and proper nutrition in promoting optimal health for both the baby and the mother. Instruction should also emphasize the importance of a woman consulting a health-care provider if she suspects she is pregnant. The harmful effects of certain substances on the fetus (e.g., alcohol, tobacco, and other drugs as well as environmental hazards, such as lead) should be emphasized, including the periods during which the fetus is most susceptible to developing birth defects. Genetic disorders and conditions can also cause birth defects. Fortunately, they can often be identified when they occur in families. Some genetic disorders are so serious that they may influence one's decision to become a parent. In that event a couple may wish to

Expressing support and compassion for others who are grieving, including allowing their friends to be sad and to express their feelings

Recognizing questions they have regarding death and dying and discussing these questions with parents, religious leaders, and other trusted adults

Reviewing family histories and determining whether a genetic disorder exists in the family

III. Expectations
and Content,
by Grade Level

High School

Unifying Idea:
An understanding of
the process of growth
and development

Grade-level concepts and content	Examples of skills and behaviors
Life cycle:	

consider adoption. Care of a newborn, including the importance of immunizations and well-baby care, may also be discussed at this time.

Because death and dying are a part of the life cycle and the death of others is a part of everyone's experience, students should have an opportunity to explore death and dying. Normal emotions associated with death and dying include fear, discomfort, concern, and nervousness. After a death and other types of loss, people may feel grief, anger, resentment, abandonment, fear, despair, pain, guilt, acceptance, or relief. In time one progresses through the mourning process, and feelings of grief usually diminish. Not everyone, however, experiences the same mourning process. The stages of the process may include denial, anger, bargaining, depression, and acceptance.

Expectation 7

Students will understand and accept individual differences in growth and development.

Grade-level concepts and content	Examples of skills and behaviors
Growth and development:	
A continuing emphasis on individual differences in physical, mental, and social growth and development is appropriate at this	▪ Demonstrating an understanding of individual differences ▪ Adapting group activities to include a variety of students

▪ Identifies previously introduced skills or behaviors that should be built on and reinforced.

Chapter 3
Health Education

III. Expectations
and Content,
by Grade Level

High School

Unifying Idea:
An understanding of
the process of growth
and development

Expectation 7 (Continued)

Grade-level concepts and content	*Examples of skills and behaviors*

Growth and development:

level. Students should understand that people experience changes and stages at their own pace.

Adolescents, especially adolescent athletes, are often preoccupied with attaining an idealized body size and shape and are particularly susceptible to nutrition quackery, eating disorders, and the lure of performance-enhancing substances, such as steroids. The curriculum should continue to emphasize the importance of basing personal nutrition and fitness plans on valid scientific data. Students need to be reminded that a wide range of body types is normal and that trying to conform to an idealized image is not only unrealistic but may be unhealthy. Desperate attempts to lose weight to conform to a culturally defined body shape and size may result in eating disorders that require professional treatment.

- Developing a realistic body image
- Recognizing health, nutrition, and psychological problems associated with not having a realistic body image, including dieting and eating disorders, and seeking appropriate help
- Recognizing the effects of performance-altering substances and avoiding the use of those substances
- Promoting acceptance of a range of body types and abilities
- Using scientific data as a basis for individual nutrition and fitness plans

Mental and emotional development:

Setting long-term goals for oneself as a way of focusing and guiding one's life can be a particularly effective strategy at this level. While acknowledging the role of heredity in growth and development, students should be encouraged to set immediate and long-term personal health and physical fitness goals. As they develop long-term goals, students should recognize that almost all

- Identifying, expressing, and managing feelings appropriately
- Developing and using effective communication skills
- Recognizing one's own strengths and limitations
- Using coping strategies, including time-management skills
- Developing a focus on the future

■ Identifies previously introduced skills or behaviors that should be built on and reinforced.

143

Chapter 3
Health Education

III. Expectations
and Content,
by Grade Level

High School

Unifying Idea:
An understanding of
the process of growth
and development

Grade-level concepts and content	Examples of skills and behaviors

Mental and emotional development:

students can expect to spend at least part of their adult lives in the work force. Increasingly, jobs and careers of every description are open to qualified persons regardless of gender.

Students should have the opportunity to explore the expectation of tragedy or loss in their lives and examine successful coping strategies. Events such as the loss of a loved one or a serious illness in the family will be experienced by most people at some point in their lives. Students can discuss coping strategies, such as receiving support from family members, drawing strength from religious beliefs, or seeking assistance from friends or a counselor, and can determine which coping strategies would be most effective in helping them through a difficult time.

Expectation 8

Students will understand their developing sexuality, will choose to abstain from sexual activity, will learn about protecting their sexual health, and will treat the sexuality of others with respect.

Grade-level concepts and content	Examples of skills and behaviors

Sexuality:

Note: The *Education Code* requires that parents be notified before human reproductive organs and their functions and processes are discussed.

A strong emphasis on abstinence should be continued at this grade span. Students should be encouraged to make a commitment to abstain

■ Developing and using effective communication skills, including the ability to discuss with parents questions regarding sexuality

■ Identifying appropriate ways to show affection

■ Identifies previously introduced skills or behaviors that should be built on and reinforced.

Chapter 3
Health Education

III. Expectations
and Content,
by Grade Level

High School

Unifying Idea:
An understanding of
the process of growth
and development

Expectation 8 (Continued)

Grade-level concepts and content	*Examples of skills and behaviors*

Sexuality:

from sexual activity until they are ready for marriage. Even those who have already engaged in sexual intercourse can choose to be abstinent. However, contraceptive methods and their relative effectiveness and ineffectiveness should be discussed. Instruction should emphasize that abstinence is the only totally effective method of contraception and that all other methods carry a risk of failure in preventing unwanted teenage pregnancy and sexually transmitted diseases. The consequences of unwanted pregnancies and the effects of teenage pregnancy on the teenagers, their child, their parents, and society should also be explored.

Students should be made aware that sexual feelings and desires are natural but that they do not have to act on those feelings. Sexual feelings, love, and intimacy are distinct aspects of sexual attraction. Responsible sexual behavior can and should be defined. Students who date should discuss limits with their dating partners and should expect those partners to respect those limits. Even when tempted to engage in sexual activity, students can exercise self-control.

A factual, substantiated discussion of homosexuality may be included at this level. (*Note:* School district governing boards considering such a discussion should refer to "Family Living" in Section II of this chapter and to Appendix A.) Students should recognize that it is a common experience to feel some affection for both

- Recognizing and avoiding situations that place one at risk of participating in sexual activity

- Avoiding, recognizing, and responding to negative social influences and pressure to become sexually active

- Demonstrating assertive and refusal skills and applying those skills to situations involving pressure to be sexually active

- Identifying ways to seek assistance if abused

- Practicing behaviors that support the decision to abstain from sexual activity, including self-control, use of reason as a basis for action, self-discipline, a sense of responsibility, religious convictions, or ethical considerations

Analyzing messages about sexuality from society, including the media, and identifying how those messages affect behavior

Evaluating what students can do to counteract the false norms portrayed in the media

■ Identifies previously introduced skills or behaviors that should be built on and reinforced.

Chapter 3
Health Education

III. Expectations
and Content,
by Grade Level

High School

Unifying Idea:
An understanding of
the process of growth
and development

Grade-level concepts and content	Examples of skills and behaviors

Sexuality:

men and women and that feelings of affection for persons of the same sex are not necessarily an indication of homosexuality. Teenagers who have questions about their sexual orientation may be reluctant to discuss the topic for fear of reprisal. Students should respect the rights of others to seek information from a parent or other trusted and knowledgeable adult. The California Student Safety and Violence Prevention Act of 2000 (AB 537) promotes an appreciation of diversity in a democratic society. Name-calling or other hurtful actions must not be tolerated. Teachers, counselors, physicians, religious leaders, and community resource centers may offer support for young people who have concerns about their sexual orientation. While respecting religious and personal beliefs, the curriculum in this content area should affirm the dignity of all people.

Physical, mental, social, and cultural factors influence attitudes and behaviors regarding sexuality. Attitudes about proper behavior for men and women differ among families and cultures. Gender stereotypes may influence behavior, career paths, relationships, and so on, but these stereotypes do not have to be accepted. Social messages about sexuality may be confusing and contradictory. False images of sexual behavior are often portrayed in the media. Students should have opportunities to explore and analyze the effects of social and cultural influences on human sexuality.

Chapter 3
Health Education

III. Expectations
and Content,
by Grade Level

High School

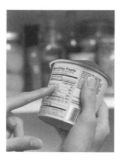

Unifying Idea
Informed use of health-related information, products, and services

Expectation:

9. Students will identify information, products, and services that may be helpful or harmful to their health.

Expectation 9

Students will identify information, products, and services that may be helpful or harmful to their health.

Grade-level concepts and content	*Examples of skills and behaviors*
	Products and services:

At this level it is especially important that students, many of whom will receive no further instruction in health education, become informed health consumers. Students' failure to become informed can have a negative influence not only on the students but on all of society as well. The health-care system is a product of our society's cumulative economic and political choices. Students can help to improve this system by becoming well-informed, careful consumers. To do so requires students to learn that there are primary points of entry for obtaining health care, including preventive, diagnostic, and treatment services, and that it is important to have an established source for primary care, rather than depend on an emergency room.

Students should be able to apply criteria for selecting health services, products, and information. For example, students might analyze

- Identifying a variety of consumer influences and analyzing how those influences affect decisions
- Recognizing helpful products and services
- Using critical-thinking skills to analyze marketing and advertising techniques and their influence on the selection of health-related services and products
- Seeking care from the nurse's office or school-linked services with their families when appropriate
- Identifying appropriate sources of health services for a variety of illnesses and being able to use those services
- Developing and applying criteria for the selection or rejection of health products, services, and information, including products or services designed to enhance physical fitness, such as exercise gear

■ Identifies previously introduced skills or behaviors that should be built on and reinforced.

147

Chapter 3
Health Education

III. Expectations
and Content,
by Grade Level

High School

Unifying Idea:
Informed use of
health-related
information,
products,
and services

Grade-level concepts and content	*Examples of skills and behaviors*

Products and services:

major types of health-insurance coverage and develop criteria for selecting health insurance. Or they might analyze how to access public and private health services by learning how to make appointments and complete health and insurance forms. The costs and benefits of health products, services, and information can also be analyzed. Students should develop strategies for identifying and combating fraudulent health products, services, and information. They should also continue to analyze the influence of advertising, especially targeted advertising, on the selection of health products and services. The legal rights of individuals to obtaining health care services should also be explored.

    Many avenues are available to students at this level for pursuing community service experiences related to health care and prevention. Voluntary health-care organizations offer one way to introduce students to educational and other resources in the community through which they can contribute to the support of community health needs.

■ Using labels to compare the contents of food products

Using critical-thinking skills to analyze the cost benefits of health care products and services

Developing and using strategies for identifying and combating fraudulent or misleading health products, services, and information

Food choices:

    As high school students become more skilled consumers, they need to be able to understand the factors that influence the cost, quality, availability, and variety of food in

■ Using critical-thinking skills to analyze marketing and advertising techniques and their influence on food selection

■ Identifies previously introduced skills or behaviors that should be built on and reinforced.

Chapter 3
Health Education

III. Expectations
and Content,
by Grade Level

High School

Unifying Idea:
Informed use of
health-related
information,
products,
and services

Expectation 9 (Continued)

Grade-level concepts and content	*Examples of skills and behaviors*

Food choices:

the marketplace locally, nationally, and internationally. To be skilled consumers, students also need to be able to evaluate nutrition information. Many nutritional claims, products, and so-called research are deceptive and can lead to serious adverse health consequences. Students need to know how and where to obtain valid, reliable information on nutrition.

■ Using valid nutrition information to make healthy food choices

■ Using unit pricing to determine the most economical purchases

■ Using effective consumer skills to purchase healthy foods within budget constraints and in a variety of settings

■ Using critical-thinking skills to distinguish facts from fallacies concerning the nutritional value of foods and food supplements

■ Adapting recipes to make them more healthy by lowering the amount of fat, salt, or sugar and increasing the amount of fiber

Using critical-thinking skills to analyze weight modification practices and selecting appropriate practices to maintain, lose, or gain weight according to individual need and scientific research

■ Identifies previously introduced skills or behaviors that should be built on and reinforced.

Scope and Sequence of Health Instruction

This section presents a summary and overview of key aspects of Chapter 3 of the *Health Framework.* Its purpose is to describe the health curriculum across the grade levels in a format that will make the key concepts more accessible to curriculum planners. The *grade-span* expectations included in the 1994 framework have been organized into *grade-level* expectations. The new chart in this section clearly indicates where the instructional emphases should be placed to achieve the overall health education expectations. The use of this chart should improve continuity and avoid duplication as students progress from one grade to the next. Each skill that should be emphasized is noted by a pyramid symbol. The content, skills, and behaviors contained in the chart are simply examples and are not intended to be comprehensive, thus offering flexibility to each school district to apply the unifying ideas and expectations to content areas as appropriate within their communities.

Although designed as a guide for curriculum planning, this section is not intended as a substitute for the careful study of the entire *Health Framework.* Rather, the purpose of this section is to simplify curriculum planning by presenting sample grade-level emphases and some of the instructional concepts and expectations of student learning explored in this chapter. In addition, curriculum planners should take into account the nine content areas of health instruction reflected in the expectations of student learning and summarized below:

- Personal Health
- Consumer and Community Health
- Injury Prevention and Safety
- Alcohol, Tobacco, and Other Drugs
- Nutrition
- Environmental Health
- Family Living
- Individual Growth and Development
- Communicable and Chronic Diseases

Although not identified specifically in the following matrix, the nine content areas are the traditional focus of health education. They are embedded in the skills and behaviors for *all* grade levels. This section provides an example of how curriculum planners might reorganize the grade-level expectations.

The following Grade-Level Emphases Chart was designed by health educators who carefully selected skills and behaviors discussed in this chapter of the framework. Each item is intended to assist teachers in helping students meet grade-level expectations. The contributing health educators, representing each of the kindergarten-through-grade-twelve levels, not only collaborated on which skills should be taught at a given grade level, but also came to consensus on the skills that students should have mastered at the previous grade level and the skills that students should master at the next grade level.

The Grade-Level Emphases Chart presents these skills and behaviors, which build sequentially, in ways that are age-appropriate. Skills and behaviors for the later grades include and build on skills and behaviors that are developed in the earlier grades.

Grade-Level Emphases Chart

Skills that should be emphasized are noted by a pyramid symbol (▲).

Kindergarten Through Grade Three

Expectation 1: Students will demonstrate ways in which they can enhance and maintain their health and well-being.

Kindergarten	Grade one	Grade two	Grade three
The Human Body			
Practice good personal hygiene.	▲ Practice good personal hygiene.	▲ Practice good personal hygiene.	▲ Practice good personal hygiene.
	▲ Use protective equipment or practice protective behaviors.	▲ Use protective equipment or practice protective behaviors.	▲ Use protective equipment or practice protective behaviors.
Food Choices			
Make healthy food choices.	Make healthy food choices.	▲ Make healthy food choices.	▲ Make healthy food choices.
Group foods in many different ways.	▲ Group foods in many different ways.	Group foods in many different ways.	▲ Group foods in many different ways.
▲ Prepare and try a variety of healthy foods.	▲ Prepare and try a variety of healthy foods.	▲ Prepare and try a variety of healthy foods.	▲ Prepare and try a variety of healthy foods.
		Analyze influences on food choices.	▲ Analyze influences on food choices.
			▲ Establish and maintain healthy eating practices.
Physical Activity			
▲ Participate regularly in active play and enjoyable physical activities.	▲ Participate regularly in active play and enjoyable physical activities.	▲ Participate regularly in active play and enjoyable physical activities.	▲ Participate regularly in active play and enjoyable physical activities.
▲ Observe safety rules during physical activities.	▲ Observe safety rules during physical activities.	▲ Observe safety rules during physical activities.	▲ Observe safety rules during physical activities.
Explore out-of-school play activities that promote fitness and health.	Explore out-of-school play activities that promote fitness and health.	Explore out-of-school play activities that promote fitness and health.	Explore out-of-school play activities that promote fitness and health.

Kindergarten Through Grade Three (Continued)

Expectation 1 (Continued)

Kindergarten	Grade one	Grade two	Grade three
Mental and Emotional Health			
▲ Identify and share feelings in appropriate ways.	▲ Identify and share feelings in appropriate ways.	▲ Identify and share feelings in appropriate ways.	▲ Identify and share feelings in appropriate ways.
▲ Avoid self-destructive behaviors and practice self-control.	▲ Avoid self-destructive behaviors and practice self-control.	Avoid self-destructive behaviors and practice self-control.	Avoid self-destructive behaviors and practice self-control.
Develop and use effective coping strategies.	Develop and use effective coping strategies.	▲ Develop and use effective coping strategies.	▲ Develop and use effective coping strategies.
Demonstrate personal characteristics that contribute to self-confidence and self-esteem.	▲ Demonstrate personal characteristics that contribute to self-confidence and self-esteem.	Demonstrate personal characteristics that contribute to self-confidence and self-esteem.	Demonstrate personal characteristics that contribute to self-confidence and self-esteem.
Develop protective factors that help foster resiliency.	Develop protective factors that help foster resiliency.	Develop protective factors that help foster resiliency.	Develop protective factors that help foster resiliency.
Develop and use effective communication skills.	Develop and use effective communication skills.	▲ Develop and use effective communication skills.	Develop and use effective communication skills.

Expectation 2: Students will understand and demonstrate behaviors that prevent disease and speed recovery from illness.

Kindergarten	Grade one	Grade two	Grade three
Disease Prevention			
Practice positive health behaviors to reduce the risk of disease.	Practice positive health behaviors to reduce the risk of disease.	Practice positive health behaviors to reduce the risk of disease.	▲ Practice positive health behaviors to reduce the risk of disease.
Prepare food as a way of learning about sanitary food preparation and storage.	Prepare food as a way of learning about sanitary food preparation and storage.	Prepare food as a way of learning about sanitary food preparation and storage.	▲ Prepare food as a way of learning about sanitary food preparation and storage.
Cooperate in regular health screenings.	Cooperate in regular health screenings.	Cooperate in regular health screenings.	Cooperate in regular health screenings.

Kindergarten Through Grade Three (Continued)

Kindergarten	Grade one	Grade two	Grade three
Treatment of Disease			
▲ Take medicines properly under the direction of parents or health-care providers.	▲ Take medicines properly under the direction of parents or health-care providers.	Take medicines properly under the direction of parents or health-care providers.	Take medicines properly under the direction of parents or health-care providers.
▲ Recognize symptoms of common illnesses.	▲ Recognize symptoms of common illnesses.	▲ Recognize symptoms of common illnesses.	▲ Recognize symptoms of common illnesses.
			Cooperate with parents and health-care providers in the treatment or management of disease.
Expectation 3: Students will practice behaviors that reduce the risk of becoming involved in potentially dangerous situations and react to potentially dangerous situations in ways that help to protect their health.			
Potentially Dangerous Situations			
▲ Practice safe behavior in or near motorized vehicles.	▲ Practice safe behavior in or near motorized vehicles.	▲ Practice safe behavior in or near motorized vehicles.	Practice safe behavior in or near motorized vehicles.
▲ Practice safe behavior in or near water.	▲ Practice safe behavior in or near water.	▲ Practice safe behavior in or near water.	Practice safe behavior in or near water.
▲ Interact safely with strangers.	▲ Interact safely with strangers.	▲ Interact safely with strangers.	▲ Interact safely with strangers.
Develop and use skills to avoid, resolve, and cope with conflicts.	Develop and use skills to avoid, resolve, and cope with conflicts.	Develop and use skills to avoid, resolve, and cope with conflicts.	▲ Develop and use skills to avoid, resolve, and cope with conflicts.
▲ Report or obtain assistance when faced with unsafe situations.	▲ Report or obtain assistance when faced with unsafe situations.	Report or obtain assistance when faced with unsafe situations.	Report or obtain assistance when faced with unsafe situations.
▲ Practice behaviors that help prevent poisonings.	▲ Practice behaviors that help prevent poisonings.	Practice behaviors that help prevent poisonings.	Practice behaviors that help prevent poisonings.
Practice safe behavior in recreational activities.	Practice safe behavior in recreational activities.	Practice safe behavior in recreational activities.	Practice safe behavior in recreational activities.
			▲ Develop and use skills to identify, avoid, and cope with potentially dangerous situations.

Kindergarten Through Grade Three (Continued)

Expectation 3 (Continued)

Alcohol, Tobacco, and Other Drugs

Kindergarten	Grade one	Grade two	Grade three
Distinguish between helpful and harmful substances.	▲ Distinguish between helpful and harmful substances.	Distinguish between helpful and harmful substances.	▲ Distinguish between helpful and harmful substances.
			Identify ways to cope with or seek assistance when confronted with situations involving alcohol, tobacco, and other drugs.
		▲ Develop and use interpersonal and communication skills.	▲ Develop and use interpersonal and communication skills.
			▲ Exercise self-control.

Child Abuse, Including Sexual Exploitation (*Penal Code 11166[a]*)

Kindergarten	Grade one	Grade two	Grade three
			Identify ways to seek assistance if worried, abused, or threatened.
▲ Develop and use communication skills to tell others when touching is unwanted.	▲ Develop and use communication skills to tell others when touching is unwanted.	▲ Develop and use communication skills to tell others when touching is unwanted.	Develop and use communication skills to tell others when touching is unwanted.

Emergencies

Kindergarten	Grade one	Grade two	Grade three
▲ Recognize emergencies and respond appropriately.	▲ Recognize emergencies and respond appropriately.	Recognize emergencies and respond appropriately.	Recognize emergencies and respond appropriately.
▲ Practice appropriate behaviors during fire drills, earthquake drills, and other disaster drills.	Practice appropriate behaviors during fire drills, earthquake drills, and other disaster drills.	Practice appropriate behaviors during fire drills, earthquake drills, and other disaster drills.	Practice appropriate behaviors during fire drills, earthquake drills, and other disaster drills.

Kindergarten Through Grade Three (Continued)

Expectation 4: Students will understand and demonstrate how to play a positive, active role in promoting the health of their families.

Kindergarten	Grade one	Grade two	Grade three
Roles of Family Members			
▲ Develop and use effective communication skills.	▲ Develop and use effective communication skills.	▲ Develop and use effective communication skills.	▲ Develop and use effective communication skills.
			Demonstrate ways to help support positive family interactions, such as listening to and following directions and showing care and concern toward other family members.
			Support and value all family members.
Change Within the Family			
Identify feelings related to changes within the family.	Identify feelings related to changes within the family.	▲ Identify feelings related to changes within the family.	▲ Identify feelings related to changes within the family.

Expectation 5: Students will understand and demonstrate how to promote positive health practices within the school and community, including how to cultivate positive relationships with their peers.

Kindergarten	Grade one	Grade two	Grade three
Friendship and Peer Relationships			
▲ Know and use appropriate ways to make new friends.	▲ Know and use appropriate ways to make new friends.	▲ Know and use appropriate ways to make new friends.	▲ Know and use appropriate ways to make new friends.
▲ Demonstrate acceptable actions toward others.	▲ Demonstrate acceptable actions toward others.	▲ Demonstrate acceptable actions toward others.	▲ Demonstrate acceptable actions toward others.
▲ Demonstrate positive ways to show or express feelings.	▲ Demonstrate positive ways to show or express feelings.	▲ Demonstrate positive ways to show or express feelings.	▲ Demonstrate positive ways to show or express feelings.
▲ Resolve conflicts in a positive, constructive way.	▲ Resolve conflicts in a positive, constructive way.	▲ Resolve conflicts in a positive, constructive way.	▲ Resolve conflicts in a positive, constructive way.
▲ Demonstrate acceptable methods of gaining attention.	▲ Demonstrate acceptable methods of gaining attention.	▲ Demonstrate acceptable methods of gaining attention.	▲ Demonstrate acceptable methods of gaining attention.

Kindergarten Through Grade Three (Continued)

Expectation 5 (Continued)

Kindergarten	Grade one	Grade two	Grade three
School and Community-Based Efforts to Promote and Protect Health			
▲ Understand and follow school rules related to health.	▲ Understand and follow school rules related to health.	▲ Understand and follow school rules related to health.	▲ Understand and follow school rules related to health.
Participate in school efforts to promote health.	Participate in school efforts to promote health.	Participate in school efforts to promote health.	Participate in school efforts to promote health.
Assume responsibility for helping to take care of the school.	Assume responsibility for helping to take care of the school.	Assume responsibility for helping to take care of the school.	Assume responsibility for helping to take care of the school.

Expectation 6: Students will understand the variety of physical, mental, emotional, and social changes that occur throughout life.

Kindergarten	Grade one	Grade two	Grade three
Life Cycle			
Describe the cycle of growth and development in humans and other animal species.	▲ Describe the cycle of growth and development in humans and other animal species.	▲ Describe the cycle of growth and development in humans and other animal species.	Demonstrate an understanding of the aging process (e.g., why older adults may have needs different from those of children).

Expectation 7: Students will understand and accept individual differences in growth and development.

Kindergarten	Grade one	Grade two	Grade three
Growth and Development			
Demonstrate an understanding of individual differences.	Demonstrate an understanding of individual differences.	Demonstrate an understanding of individual differences.	▲ Demonstrate an understanding of individual differences.
▲ Adapt group activities to include a variety of students.	▲ Adapt group activities to include a variety of students.	▲ Adapt group activities to include a variety of students.	▲ Adapt group activities to include a variety of students.

Kindergarten Through Grade Three (Continued)

157

Kindergarten	Grade one	Grade two	Grade three
Mental and Emotional Development			
Identify, express, and manage feelings appropriately.	Identify, express, and manage feelings appropriately.	Identify, express, and manage feelings appropriately.	Identify, express, and manage feelings appropriately.
Develop and use effective communication skills.	Develop and use effective communication skills.	Develop and use effective communication skills.	Develop and use effective communication skills.
Expectation 8: Students will identify information, products, and services that may be helpful or harmful to their health.			
Products and Services			
▲ Identify health care workers.	▲ Identify health care workers.		
	Identify a variety of consumer influences and analyze how those influences affect decisions.	▲ Identify a variety of consumer influences and analyze how those influences affect decisions.	▲ Identify a variety of consumer influences and analyze how those influences affect decisions.
			Identify places for obtaining health and social services and learn what types of services are provided.
Products and Services/Food Choices			
			Read and interpret information available on food labels.
			Use labels to compare the contents of food products.
			Identify ads and recognize strategies used to influence decisions.
			Practice various positive responses to those influences.

Grades Four Through Six

Expectation 1: Students will demonstrate ways in which they can enhance and maintain their health and well-being.

Grade Four	Grade Five	Grade Six
The Human Body		
▲ Practice good personal hygiene, with particular attention to the changing needs of preadolescents and adolescents.	▲ Practice good personal hygiene, with particular attention to the changing needs of preadolescents and adolescents.	▲ Practice good personal hygiene, with particular attention to the changing needs of preadolescents and adolescents.
Use protective equipment or practice protective behaviors.	Use protective equipment or practice protective behaviors.	Use protective equipment or practice protective behaviors.
Food Choices		
▲ Establish and maintain healthy eating practices.	▲ Establish and maintain healthy eating practices.	▲ Establish and maintain healthy eating practices.
Make healthy food choices.	Make healthy food choices.	Make healthy food choices.
Prepare a variety of healthy foods.	Prepare a variety of healthy foods.	
		Analyze influences on food choices.
Practice kitchen safety.	Practice kitchen safety.	Practice kitchen safety.
Physical Activity		
▲ Participate regularly in a variety of enjoyable physical activities.	▲ Participate regularly in a variety of enjoyable physical activities.	▲ Participate regularly in a variety of enjoyable physical activities.
▲ Set personal fitness goals.	▲ Set personal fitness goals.	▲ Set personal fitness goals.
▲ Explore out-of-school play activities that promote fitness and health.	▲ Explore out-of-school play activities that promote fitness and health.	▲ Explore out-of-school play activities that promote fitness and health.
▲ Obtain a sufficient amount of sleep.	▲ Obtain a sufficient amount of sleep.	▲ Obtain a sufficient amount of sleep.
	Observe safety rules during physical activities.	Observe safety rules during physical activities.

Grades Four Through Six (Continued)

Mental and Emotional Health

Grade Four	Grade Five	Grade Six
▲ Demonstrate personal characteristics that contribute to self-confidence and self-esteem.	Demonstrate personal characteristics that contribute to self-confidence and self-esteem.	Demonstrate personal characteristics that contribute to self-confidence and self-esteem.
Develop and use effective communication skills.	▲ Develop and use effective communication skills.	▲ Develop and use effective communication skills.
	▲ Develop and use effective coping strategies.	▲ Develop and use effective coping strategies.
▲ Identify and share feelings in appropriate ways.	Identify and share feelings in appropriate ways.	Identify and share feelings in appropriate ways.
		Develop protective factors that help foster resiliency.
		Avoid self-destructive behaviors and practice strategies for resisting negative peer pressure.

Expectation 2: Students will understand and demonstrate behaviors that prevent disease and speed recovery from illness.

Disease Prevention

Grade Four	Grade Five	Grade Six
Practice positive health behaviors to reduce the risk of disease.	Practice positive health behaviors to reduce the risk of disease.	▲ Practice positive health behaviors to reduce the risk of disease.
Practice good personal hygiene.	Practice good personal hygiene.	Practice good personal hygiene.
		Cooperate in regular health screenings.
		Demonstrate care and concern toward ill persons in the family, the school, and the community.

Grades Four Through Six (Continued)

Expectation 2 (Continued)

Grade Four	Grade Five	Grade Six
Treatment of Disease		
▲ Recognize symptoms of common illnesses.	Recognize symptoms of common illnesses.	Recognize symptoms of common illnesses.
		Take prescription and over-the-counter medicines properly.
Cooperate with parents and health care providers in the treatment or management of disease.	Cooperate with parents and health care providers in the treatment or management of disease.	Cooperate with parents and health care providers in the treatment or management of disease.
		Interpret correctly instructions for taking medicine.

Expectation 3: Students will practice behaviors that reduce the risk of becoming involved in potentially dangerous situations and react to potentially dangerous situations in ways that help to protect their health.

Potentially Dangerous Situations

Grade Four	Grade Five	Grade Six
▲ Develop and use skills to avoid, resolve, and cope with conflicts.	▲ Develop and use skills to avoid, resolve, and cope with conflicts.	▲ Develop and use skills to avoid, resolve, and cope with conflicts.
Develop and use skills to identify, avoid, and cope with potentially dangerous situations.	▲ Develop and use skills to identify, avoid, and cope with potentially dangerous situations.	▲ Develop and use skills to identify, avoid, and cope with potentially dangerous situations.
Understand and follow rules prohibiting possession of weapons at school.	▲ Understand and follow rules prohibiting possession of weapons at school.	▲ Understand and follow rules prohibiting possession of weapons at school.
		Practice safe behavior in or near motorized vehicles.
		Practice safe behavior in recreational activities.
		Practice safe behavior in and near water.
		Report or obtain assistance when faced with unsafe situations.

Grades Four Through Six (Continued)

Grade Four	Grade Five	Grade Six
Alcohol, Tobacco, and Other Drugs		
▲ Distinguish between helpful and harmful substances.	Distinguish between helpful and harmful substances.	Distinguish between helpful and harmful substances.
	▲ Avoid, recognize, and respond to negative social influences and pressures to use alcohol, tobacco, or other drugs.	▲ Avoid, recognize, and respond to negative social influences and pressures to use alcohol, tobacco, or other drugs.
		Exercise self-control.
		Develop and use interpersonal and communication skills.
Identify ways to cope with or seek assistance when confronted with situations involving alcohol, tobacco, and other drugs.	▲ Identify ways to cope with or seek assistance when confronted with situations involving alcohol, tobacco, and other drugs.	Identify ways to cope with or seek assistance when confronted with situations involving alcohol, tobacco, and other drugs.
▲ Identify ways of obtaining help to resist pressure to use alcohol, tobacco, or other drugs.	Identify ways of obtaining help to resist pressure to use alcohol, tobacco, or other drugs.	Identify ways of obtaining help to resist pressure to use alcohol, tobacco, or other drugs.
		Differentiate between the use and misuse of prescription and nonprescription drugs.
		Use positive peer pressure to help counteract the negative effects of living in an environment where alcohol, tobacco, or other drug abuse or dependency exists.
Child Abuse, Including Sexual Exploitation (Penal Code 11166[a])		
Identify ways to seek assistance if worried, abused, or threatened.	Identify ways to seek assistance if worried, abused or threatened.	Identify ways to seek assistance if worried, abused, or threatened.
		Recognize and avoid situations that can increase risk of abuse.

Grades Four Through Six (Continued)

Expectation 3 (Continued)

Grade Four	Grade Five	Grade Six
Emergencies		
Recognize emergencies and respond appropriately, including knowing where to find emergency supplies.	Recognize emergencies and respond appropriately, including knowing where to find emergency supplies.	▲ Recognize emergencies and respond appropriately, including (1) knowing where to find emergency supplies; (2) demonstrating proficiency in basic first-aid procedures; and (3) using precautions when dealing with other people's blood.
▲ Understand the family emergency plan.	Understand the family emergency plan.	Understand the family emergency plan.

Expectation 4: Students will understand and demonstrate how to play a positive, active role in promoting the health of their families.

Grade Four	Grade Five	Grade Six
Roles of Family Members		
Demonstrate ways to help support positive family interactions.	Demonstrate ways to help support positive family interactions.	Demonstrate ways to help support positive family interactions.
Practice health-promoting behaviors with the family.	Practice health-promoting behaviors with the family.	Practice health-promoting behaviors with the family.
		Participate in daily activities that help maintain the family.
		Support and value all family members.
		Develop and use effective communication skills.
Change Within the Family		
		Identify and effectively express feelings related to changes within the family.
		Use effective strategies to cope with changes within the family, including identifying a support system.

Grades Four Through Six (Continued)

Expectation 5: Students will understand and demonstrate how to promote positive health practices within the school and community, including how to cultivate positive relationships with their peers.

Grade Four	Grade Five	Grade Six
Friendship and Peer Relationships		
Know and use appropriate ways to make new friends.	Know and use appropriate ways to make new friends.	Know and use appropriate ways to make new friends.
▲ Resolve conflicts in a positive, constructive way.	▲ Resolve conflicts in a positive, constructive way.	Resolve conflicts in a positive, constructive way.
Demonstrate positive actions toward others.	▲ Demonstrate positive actions toward others.	Demonstrate positive actions toward others.
	▲ Demonstrate acceptable methods of gaining attention.	Demonstrate acceptable methods of gaining attention.
	Demonstrate acceptable ways to show or express feelings.	Demonstrate acceptable ways to show or express feelings.
	▲ Demonstrate how to resist negative peer pressure.	▲ Demonstrate how to resist negative peer pressure.
School and Community-Based Efforts to Promote and Protect Health		
Participate in school efforts to promote health.	Participate in school efforts to promote health.	▲ Participate in school efforts to promote health.
Participate in community efforts to address local health and environmental issues.	Participate in community efforts to address local health and environmental issues.	▲ Participate in community efforts to address local health and environmental issues.
Understand and follow school rules related to health.	Understand and follow school rules related to health.	▲ Understand and follow school rules related to health.
		Assume responsibility for helping to take care of the school.
		Contribute to the strengthening of health-related policies at school.
		Recognize that public policies and laws influence health-related issues.

Grades Four Through Six (Continued)

Expectation 6: Students will understand the variety of physical, mental, emotional, and social changes that occur throughout life.

Life Cycle

Grade Four	Grade Five	Grade Six
Recognize the changes that occur during preadolescence.	▲ Recognize the changes that occur during preadolescence.	▲ Recognize the changes that occur during preadolescence.
	▲ Use correct terminology for body parts.	▲ Use correct terminology for body parts.
	Recognize changing emotions.	Recognize changing emotions.
		▲ Develop and use effective communication skills to discuss with parents or other trusted adults the changes that occur during preadolescence.
Practice good personal hygiene.	▲ Practice good personal hygiene.	▲ Practice good personal hygiene.
Manage feelings appropriately.	Manage feelings appropriately.	Manage feelings appropriately.

Expectation 7: Students will understand and accept individual differences in growth and development.

Growth and Development

Grade Four	Grade Five	Grade Six
▲ Demonstrate an understanding of individual differences.		▲ Demonstrate an understanding of individual differences.
	Develop a realistic body image.	▲ Develop a realistic body image.
		Recognize problems associated with not having a realistic body image.
Adapt group activities to include a variety of students.	Adapt group activities to include a variety of students.	Adapt group activities to include a variety of students.

Grades Four Through Six (Continued)

Grade Four	Grade Five	Grade Six
Mental and Emotional Development		
Identify, express, and manage feelings appropriately.	Identify, express, and manage feelings appropriately.	Identify, express, and manage feelings appropriately.
Develop and use effective communication skills.	Develop and use effective communication skills.	Develop and use effective communication skills.
Develop and use strategies, including critical thinking, decision making, goal setting, and problem solving.	Develop and use strategies, including critical thinking, decision making, goal setting, and problem solving.	Develop and use strategies, including critical thinking, decision making, goal setting, and problem solving.
		Recognize one's own strengths and limitations.
		Focus on the future (e.g., realistic short-term and long-term goals).
Expectation 8: Students will identify information, products, and services that may be helpful or harmful to their health.		
Products and Services		
▲ Use critical-thinking skills to analyze marketing and advertising techniques and their influence.	▲ Use critical-thinking skills to analyze marketing and advertising techniques and their influence.	▲ Use critical-thinking skills to analyze marketing and advertising techniques and their influence.
Recognize helpful products and services.	Recognize helpful products and services.	Recognize helpful products and services.
	Identify a variety of consumer influences and analyze how those influences affect decisions.	Identify a variety of consumer influences and analyze how those influences affect decisions.
		Identify places for obtaining health and social services and learn what types of services are provided.
Identify health-care workers.		
Seek care from the school nurse or others (e.g., when needed for proper management of asthma).	Seek care from the school nurse or others (e.g., when needed for proper management of asthma).	Seek care from the school nurse or others (e.g., when needed for proper management of asthma).
		Discuss home care with parents when appropriate.

Grades Four Through Six (Continued)

Expectation 8 (Continued)

Grade Four	Grade Five	Grade Six
	Food Choices	
▲ Develop basic food-preparation skills.	▲ Develop basic food-preparation skills.	▲ Develop basic food-preparation skills.
Read and interpret information available on food labels.	Read and interpret information available on food labels.	Read and interpret information available on food labels.
Use valid nutrition information to make healthy food choices.	Use valid nutrition information to make healthy food choices.	Use valid nutrition information to make healthy food choices.
	Use critical-thinking skills to analyze marketing and advertising techniques and their influence on food selection.	Use critical-thinking skills to analyze marketing and advertising techniques and their influence on food selection.
	Use unit pricing to determine the most economical purchases.	Use unit pricing to determine the most economical purchases.
		Use labels to compare the contents of food products.
		Purchase nutritious foods in a variety of settings.
		Analyze and taste foods from different ethnic and cultural groups.

Middle School

Expectation I: Students will demonstrate ways in which they can enhance and maintain their health and well-being.

The Human Body

▲ Practice good personal hygiene, including accepting responsibility for making those behaviors part of a normal routine.

▲ Recognize and accept differences in body types and maturation levels.

Recognize and avoid potentially harmful environmental conditions, such as exposure to pesticides or lead paint.

Use protective equipment, such as wearing goggles to protect the eyes when appropriate, or practice behaviors to protect the body, such as applying sunscreen, exercising, or making healthy food choices.

Food Choices

▲ Make healthy food choices in a variety of settings.

▲ Compare caloric values of foods according to the percentage of fat, protein, and carbohydrate they contain.

▲ Establish and maintain healthy eating practices.

Select appropriate practices to maintain, lose, or gain weight according to individual needs and scientific research.

Prepare a variety of healthy foods.

Analyze influences on food choices.

Physical Activity

▲ Observe safety rules during physical activities.

▲ Develop and initiate a personal fitness plan.

Obtain a sufficient amount of sleep.

Explore ways to engage in out-of-school activities that promote fitness and health.

Participate regularly in a variety of enjoyable physical activities.

Mental and Emotional Health

Demonstrate characteristics that contribute to self-confidence and self-esteem.

Develop and use effective communication skills.

Manage strong feelings and boredom.

Develop protective factors that help foster resiliency.

Middle School (Continued)

Expectation 1—Mental and Emotional Health (Continued)

Develop and use effective coping strategies, emphasizing coping with feelings of inadequacy, sadness.

Avoid self-destructive behaviors.

Practice strategies for resisting negative peer pressure.

Identify risk factors for negative behaviors and develop effective strategies for counteracting these risk factors.

Select entertainment that promotes mental and physical health.

Expectation 2: Students will understand and demonstrate behaviors that prevent disease and speed recovery from illness.

Disease Prevention

◄ Practice good personal hygiene.

◄ Practice positive health behaviors to reduce the risk of disease.

◄ Cooperate in regular health screenings.

Practice and use effective self-examination procedures.

Demonstrate care and concern toward ill persons in the family, the school, and the community.

Make a commitment to abstain from sexual activity.

Receive and understand statistics based on the latest medical information citing the failure and success rates of condoms in preventing AIDS and other sexually transmitted diseases.

Treatment of Disease

Recognize symptoms of common illnesses.

Take prescription and over-the-counter medicines properly.

Interpret correctly instructions written on medicine container labels, including information about side effects.

Determine when treatment of illness at home is appropriate and when and how to seek further help when needed.

Accept responsibility for active involvement in the treatment or management of disease.

Middle School (Continued)

Expectation 3: Students will practice behaviors that reduce the risk of becoming involved in potentially dangerous situations and react to potentially dangerous situations in ways that help to protect their health.

Potentially Dangerous Situations

◀ Develop and use skills to identify, avoid, and cope with potentially dangerous situations.

◀ Use skills to avoid, resolve, and cope with conflicts.

◀ Understand and follow rules prohibiting possession of weapons at school.

◀ Identify risk factors that reduce risks of accidents.

◀ Practice safe behavior in or near motorized vehicles.

◀ Practice safe behavior in recreational activities, even in the absence of adults

◀ Practice safe behavior in and near water.

◀ Report or obtain assistance when faced with unsafe situations.

◀ Identify environmental factors that affect health and safety.

◀ Demonstrate how peers can help each other avoid and cope with potentially dangerous situations in healthy ways.

◀ Use thinking and decision-making skills in high-risk situations involving the use of motor vehicles and other hazardous activities.

◀ Recognize that the use of alcohol and other drugs plays a role in many dangerous situations.

Alcohol, Tobacco, and Other Drugs

◀ Develop and use interpersonal and communication skills (e.g., assertiveness, refusal, negotiation, and conflict resolution).

◀ Differentiate between the use and misuse of prescription and nonprescription drugs.

◀ Avoid, recognize, and respond to negative social influences and pressure to use alcohol, tobacco, or other drugs.

◀ Identify ways of obtaining help to resist pressure to use alcohol, tobacco, or other drugs.

◀ Identify and participate in positive alternative activities, such as alcohol-, tobacco-, and drug-free events.

◀ Exercise self-control.

◀ Distinguish between helpful and harmful substances.

◀ Use positive peer pressure to help counteract the negative effects of living in an environment where alcohol, tobacco, or other drug abuse or dependency exists.

Middle School (Continued)

Expectation 3 (Continued)

Child Abuse, Including Sexual Exploitation (*Penal Code 11166[a]*)

▲ Recognize and avoid situations that can increase risk of abuse.

Identify ways to seek assistance if worried, abused, or threatened.

Avoid, recognize, and respond to negative social influences and pressure to become sexually active, including applying refusal skills when appropriate.

Emergencies

▲ Recognize emergencies and respond appropriately, including demonstrating proficiency in basic first-aid procedures.

Develop and maintain with other family members a personal and family emergency plan, including maintaining supplies for emergencies.

Expectation 4: Students will understand and demonstrate how to play a positive, active role in promoting the health of their families.

Roles of Family Members

▲ Demonstrate ways to help support positive family interactions.

▲ Develop and use effective communication skills, including talking openly and honestly with parents when problems arise and discussing with parents questions about sexuality.

▲ Practice health-promoting behaviors within the family.

Support and value all family members.

Complete self-initiated activities beyond assigned chores to help support the family.

Identify safety hazards in the home and help to remove them.

Change Within the Family

▲ Use effective strategies to cope with change within the family, such as seeking assistance from a parent, a trusted adult, a support system, or counseling when needed.

Middle School (Continued)

Expectation 5: Students will understand and demonstrate how to promote positive health practices within the school and community, including how to cultivate positive relationships with their peers.

Friendship and Peer Relationships

◀ Know and use appropriate ways to make new friends.

◀ Demonstrate positive actions toward others.

◀ Resolve conflicts in a positive, constructive way.

◀ Demonstrate how to resist negative peer pressure.

◀ Avoid demeaning statements directed toward others.

◀ Interact effectively with many different people.

◀ Promote positive health behaviors among peers.

◀ Demonstrate acceptable methods of gaining attention.

◀ Demonstrate acceptable ways to show or express feelings.

◀ Help peers know when they should seek help from a parent or other trusted adult.

School and Community-Based Efforts to Promote and Protect Health

◀ Understand and follow school rules related to health.

◀ Participate in school efforts to promote health.

◀ Assume responsibility for helping to take care of the school.

◀ Participate in community efforts to address local health and environmental issues.

◀ Encourage others to become involved in health-promotion efforts at school.

◀ Analyze the impact of laws, policies, and practices on health-related issues.

◀ Encourage others to become involved in health-promotion efforts at many different levels.

◀ Access appropriately services available within the community.

◀ Contribute to the strengthening of health-related policies at school.

Middle School (Continued)

Expectation 6: Students will understand the variety of physical, mental, emotional, and social changes that occur throughout life.

Life Cycle

◄ Practice good personal hygiene, paying particular attention to the changing needs of adolescents.

◄ Manage feelings appropriately.

◄ Develop and use effective communication skills to discuss with parents or other trusted adults the changes that occur during adolescence.

Recognize fluctuations in emotions.

Practice behaviors that will provide the option of healthy parenting later in life, such as avoidance of substance abuse.

Expectation 7: Students will understand and accept individual differences in growth and development.

Growth and Development

◄ Demonstrate an understanding of individual differences.

◄ Develop a realistic body image.

Recognize problems associated with not having a realistic body image.

◄ Recognize the effects of performance-altering substances and avoid the use of those substances.

Adapt group activities to include a variety of students.

Mental and Emotional Development

◄ Identify, express, and manage feelings appropriately.

◄ Develop and use effective communication skills.

◄ Use coping strategies, including time-management skills.

Recognize one's own strengths and limitations.

Develop a focus on the future.

Expectation 8: Students will understand their developing sexuality, will choose to abstain from sexual activity, will learn about protecting their sexual health, and will treat the sexuality of others with respect.

Sexuality

◄ Develop and use effective communication skills, including the ability to discuss with parents questions on sexuality.

◄ Identify appropriate ways to show affection.

Middle School (Continued)

▲ Use good judgment to recognize and avoid situations that could lead to subsequent sexual activity.

▲ Practice behaviors that support the decision to abstain from sexual activity.

▲ Demonstrate assertive and refusal skills and apply those skills to situations involving pressure to be sexually active.

Avoid, recognize, and respond to negative social influences and pressure to become sexually active.

Identify ways to seek assistance if abused.

Receive and understand statistics based on the latest medical information citing the failure and success rates of condoms and other contraceptives in preventing pregnancy and sexually transmitted diseases.

Expectation 9: Students will identify information, products, and services that may be helpful or harmful to their health.

Products and Services/Food Choices

▲ Identify a variety of consumer influences and analyze how those influences affect decisions.

▲ Use critical-thinking skills to analyze marketing and advertising techniques and their influence.

▲ Identify appropriate sources of health services for a variety of illnesses.

▲ Develop and apply criteria for the selection or rejection of health products, services, and information.

Recognize helpful products and services.

Seek care from the school nurse or school-linked services when appropriate.

▲ Use critical-thinking skills to analyze marketing and advertising techniques and their influence on food selection.

Use labels to compare the contents of food products.

Use valid nutrition information to make healthy food choices.

Use unit pricing to determine the most economical purchases.

Develop basic food-preparation skills, including sanitary food preparation and storage.

Use effective consumer skills to purchase healthy foods within budget constraints.

Use critical-thinking skills to distinguish facts from fallacies concerning the nutritional value of foods.

Adapt recipes to make them more healthy by lowering fat, salt, or sugar and increasing fiber.

Use critical-thinking skills to analyze weight modification practices and select appropriate practices to maintain, lose, or gain weight.

High School

Expectation 1: Students will demonstrate ways in which they can enhance and maintain their health and well-being.

The Human Body

Practice good personal hygiene.

Use protective equipment, such as wearing a helmet when cycling, or practice behaviors to protect the body, such as avoiding exposure to excessive noises.

Recognize and accept differences in body types and maturation levels.

Respond appropriately to the physical development of older adolescents in ways that promote physical health through such preventive measures as healthy food choices and exercise.

Food Choices

◀ Make healthy food choices in a variety of settings.

◀ Establish and maintain healthy eating practices.

Select appropriate practices to maintain, lose, or gain weight based on scientific research.

◀ Recognize the need for updating one's personal nutrition plan as individual needs or activities change.

◀ Analyze influences on food choices.

Physical Activity

Observe safety rules during physical activities.

◀ Participate regularly in a variety of enjoyable physical activities.

◀ Analyze personal motivators related to pursuing physical activity.

◀ Explore ways to continue regular exercise practices when schedules change, such as during travel or while working.

Explore ways to engage in out-of-school activities that promote fitness and health.

Follow through with a personal fitness plan based on fitness goals and the results of periodic self-assessment.

Make adjustments needed for successful implementation of a personal fitness plan.

High School (Continued)

Mental and Emotional Health

▲ Demonstrate characteristics that contribute to self-confidence and self-esteem.

▲ Develop and use effective communication skills.

▲ Develop and use effective coping strategies.

▲ Avoid self-destructive behaviors and practice strategies for resisting negative peer pressure.

▲ Relate in positive ways to peers and adults in and out of school.

▲ Identify risk factors for negative behaviors and develop effective strategies for counteracting these risk factors.

Develop protective factors that help foster resiliency.

Select entertainment that promotes mental and physical health.

Identify personal habits influencing mental and emotional health and develop strategies for changing behaviors as needed to promote positive mental and emotional health.

Expectation 2: Students will understand and demonstrate behaviors that prevent disease and speed recovery from illness.

Disease Prevention

▲ Practice positive health behaviors to reduce the risk of disease.

▲ Cooperate in regular health screenings.

▲ Practice and use effective self-examination procedures.

▲ Analyze personal behaviors in relation to health, well-being, and personal goals.

Practice good personal hygiene.

Recognize the importance of prenatal and perinatal care.

Demonstrate care and concern toward ill persons in the family, the school, and the community.

Make a commitment to abstain from sexual activity.

Receive and understand statistics based on the latest medical information citing the failure and success rates of condoms in preventing AIDS and other sexually transmitted diseases.

High School (Continued)

Expectation 2 (Continued)

Treatment of Disease

▲ Recognize symptoms of common illnesses.

Take prescription and over-the-counter medicines properly.

Interpret correctly instructions written on medicine container labels, including information about side effects.

Determine when treatment of illness at home is appropriate and when and how to seek further help when needed.

Accept responsibility for active involvement in the treatment or management of disease.

Interpret correctly information provided by health-care providers regarding tests or procedures.

Analyze one's patterns related to treatment of disease to determine their effectiveness.

Expectation 3: Students will practice behaviors that reduce the risk of becoming involved in potentially dangerous situations and react to potentially dangerous situations in ways that help to protect their health.

Potentially Dangerous Situations

▲ Develop and use skills to identify, avoid, and cope with potentially dangerous situations.

▲ Use skills to avoid, resolve, and cope with conflicts.

▲ Understand and follow rules prohibiting possession of weapons at school.

▲ Identify factors that reduce risks of accidents.

▲ Recognize that the use of alcohol, tobacco, and other drugs plays a role in many dangerous situations.

▲ Use thinking and decision-making skills in high-risk situations involving motor vehicles and other safety hazards.

▲ Practice safe behavior in or near motorized vehicles, including observing basic traffic safety rules when driving, developing proficiency in handling a vehicle in difficult situations, wearing a seat belt, and ensuring that others wear seat belts.

Carry appropriate emergency equipment and use latex gloves when assisting individuals who are injured.

Practice safe behavior in recreational activities, even in the absence of adults.

Practice safe behavior in and near water.

Report or obtain assistance when faced with unsafe situations.

Identify environmental factors that affect health and safety.

Demonstrate how peers can help each other avoid and cope with potentially dangerous situations in healthy ways.

High School (Continued)

Alcohol, Tobacco, and Other Drugs

▲ Exercise self-control.

▲ Develop and use interpersonal and communication skills such as assertiveness, refusal, negotiation, and conflict resolution.

▲ Avoid, recognize, and respond to negative social influences and pressure to use alcohol, tobacco, or other drugs.

▲ Use positive peer pressure to help counteract the negative effects of living in an environment where alcohol, tobacco, or other drug abuse or dependency exists.

▲ Identify ways of obtaining help to resist pressure to use alcohol, tobacco, or other drugs.

Distinguish between helpful and harmful substances.

Differentiate between the use and misuse of prescription and nonprescription drugs.

Identify and participate in positive alternative activities, such as alcohol-, tobacco-, and drug-free events.

Help to develop and support the school's no-use policy and work to support it.

Child Abuse, Including Sexual Exploitation (*Penal Code 11166[a]*)

▲ Identify ways to seek assistance if worried, abused, or threatened.

▲ Avoid, recognize, and respond to negative social influences and pressure to become sexually active, including applying refusal skills when appropriate.

Recognize and avoid situations that can increase risk of abuse.

Develop and use assertiveness skills and learn self-defense techniques.

Emergencies

▲ Recognize emergencies and respond appropriately.

Develop and maintain with other family members a personal and family emergency plan and emergency supplies at home and in vehicles.

Identify appropriate use of local emergency services.

Use latex gloves when assisting persons who are injured.

High School (Continued)

Expectation 4: Students will understand and demonstrate how to play a positive, active role in promoting the health of their families.

Roles of Family Members

◄ Develop and use effective communication skills.

◄ Seek assistance if living in a family where abuse of alcohol or other drugs exists (e.g., participating in a support group for teens who are the children of alcoholics).

Support and value all family members.

Demonstrate ways to help support positive family interactions.

Practice health-promoting behaviors within the family.

Complete self-initiated activities beyond assigned chores to help support the family.

Identify safety hazards in the home and help to remove them.

Change Within the Family

Use effective strategies to cope with change within the family.

Develop a plan to facilitate transition from the role of a child to the role of an independent adult.

Discuss with parents plans to continue education beyond high school and develop a mutual understanding of how this will affect family roles and interactions.

Expectation 5: Students will understand and demonstrate how to promote positive health practices within the school and community, including how to cultivate positive relationships with their peers.

Friendship and Peer Relationships

◄ Know and use appropriate ways to make new friends.

◄ Demonstrate positive actions toward others.

◄ Resolve conflicts in a positive, constructive way.

◄ Interact effectively with many different people, including males and females and members of different ethnic and cultural groups.

◄ Analyze appropriate behaviors in a dating relationship.

High School (Continued)

Demonstrate how to resist negative peer pressure.

Avoid demeaning statements directed toward others.

Promote positive health behaviors among peers.

Participate in group activities as a means of getting to know other people.

Respect the dignity of others.

Respect marriage.

School and Community-Based Efforts to Promote and Protect Health

Understand and follow school rules related to health.

Participate in school efforts to promote health.

Assume responsibility for helping to take care of the school.

Participate in community efforts to address local health and environmental issues.

Encourage others to become involved in health-promotion efforts at school.

Analyze the impact of laws, policies, and practices on health-related issues.

Encourage others to become involved in health-promotion efforts at many different levels.

Access appropriately services available within the community.

Initiate and involve others in health-promotion efforts at school or in the community.

Expectation 6: Students will understand the variety of physical, mental, emotional, and social changes that occur throughout life.

Life Cycle

▲ Practice behaviors that will provide the option of healthy parenting later in life, such as avoidance of substance abuse.

▲ Recognize and be prepared to adapt to the changes that occur during life, such as changes associated with young adulthood, pregnancy, middle age, or old age.

Develop and use effective communication skills to discuss with parents or other trusted adults the changes that occur during adolescence.

Recognize and acknowledge that different people progress through different stages of the life cycle at different rates.

High School (Continued)

Expectation 6—Life Cycle (Continued)

Express support and compassion for others who are grieving.

Recognize and discuss with parents and other trusted adults questions regarding death and dying.

Review family histories and determine whether a genetic disorder exists in the family.

Expectation 7: Students will understand and accept individual differences in growth and development.

Growth and Development

▲ Demonstrate an understanding of individual differences.

▲ Develop a realistic body image.

Recognize problems associated with not having a realistic body image.

▲ Recognize the effects of performance-altering substances and avoid the use of those substances.

Adapt group activities to include a variety of students.

Promote acceptance of a range of body types and abilities.

Use scientific data as a basis for individual nutrition and fitness plans.

Mental and Emotional Development

▲ Identify, express, and manage feelings appropriately.

▲ Develop and use effective communication skills.

Recognize one's own strengths and limitations.

Use coping strategies, including time-management skills.

Develop a focus on the future.

Expectation 8: Students will understand their developing sexuality, will choose to abstain from sexual activity, will learn about protecting their sexual health, and will treat the sexuality of others with respect.

Sexuality

▲ Use good judgment to recognize and avoid situations that could lead to subsequent sexual activity.

▲ Avoid, recognize, and respond to negative social influences and pressure to become sexually active.

High School (Continued)

▲ Demonstrate assertiveness and refusal skills and apply those skills to situations involving pressure to be sexually active.

▲ Practice behaviors that support the decision to abstain from sexual activity.

▲ Analyze messages about sexuality from society, including the media, and identify how those messages affect behavior.

▲ Develop and use effective communication skills, including the ability to discuss with parents questions on sexuality.

Identify appropriate ways to show affection.

Identify ways to seek assistance if abused.

Evaluate what students can do to counteract the false norms portrayed in the media.

Receive and understand statistics based on the latest medical information citing the failure and success rates of condoms and other contraceptives in preventing pregnancy and sexually transmitted diseases.

Expectation 9: Students will identify information, products, and services that may be helpful or harmful to their health.

Products and Services/Food Choices

▲ Identify a variety of consumer influences and analyze how those influences affect decisions.

▲ Use critical-thinking skills to analyze marketing and advertising techniques and their influence.

Recognize helpful products and services.

Seek care from the school nurse or school-linked services when appropriate.

Identify appropriate sources of health services for a variety of illnesses.

Develop and apply criteria for the selection or rejection of health products, services, and information.

Use critical-thinking skills to analyze the cost benefits of health care products and services.

Develop and use strategies for identifying and combating fraudulent or misleading health products, services, and information.

▲ Use critical-thinking skills to analyze marketing and advertising techniques and their influence on food selection.

▲ Use valid nutrition information to make healthy food choices.

▲ Use critical-thinking skills to distinguish facts from fallacies concerning the nutritional value of foods and food supplements.

High School (Continued)

Expectation 9—Products and Services/Food Choices (Continued)

▲ Use critical-thinking skills to analyze weight modification practices and select appropriate practices to maintain, lose, or gain weight according to individual need and scientific research.

Use labels to compare the contents of food products.

Use unit pricing to determine the most economical purchases.

Use effective consumer skills to purchase healthy foods.

Adapt recipes to make them more healthy by lowering the amount of fat, salt, or sugar and increasing the amount of fiber.

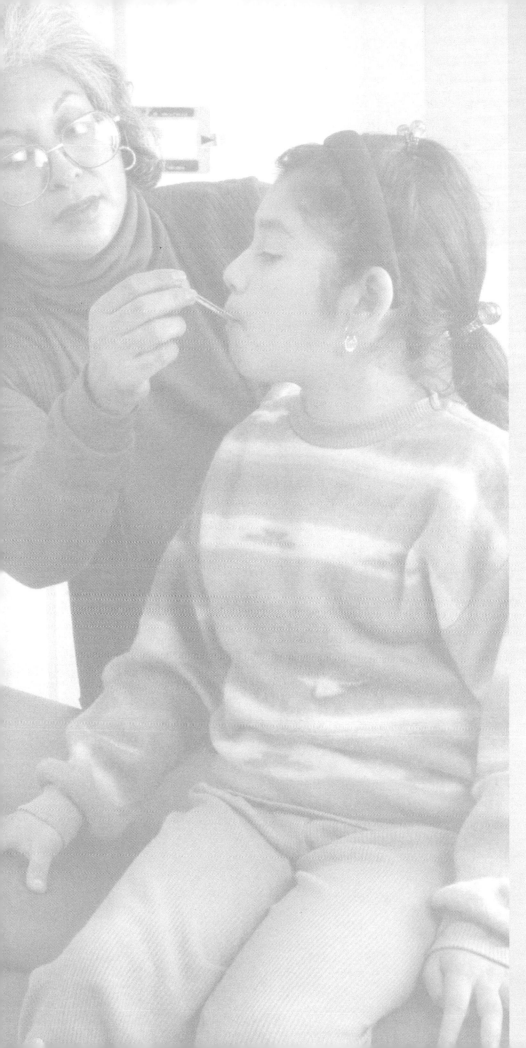

CHAPTER 4

Beyond
Health
Education

Central to an effective coordinated school health system is a carefully planned approach to developing and reinforcing health literacy in students. Health education and the coordinated school health system offer abundant opportunities for everyone in the school and the community to become involved in a collaborative undertaking. This chapter offers a variety of ways in which that reinforcement and involvement can take place.

The participation of a wide range of adults in the school and the community is an essential element of a successful coordinated school health system. The principal, the faculty, the support staff, the parents—everyone in the school—must recognize children's health as an important priority. A schoolwide focus on health ensures that emphasis will be placed on developing and sustaining healthy behaviors. If the environment of the school and the community does not reinforce healthy behaviors and choices, students may perceive that such behaviors and choices are not uniformly valued. For example, although students may, through the health curriculum, learn about the importance of a balanced diet, their behavior may be undermined by the easy availability of nonnutritious foods in hallway vending machines or at school-sponsored activities. Similarly, although the importance of regular aerobic physical activity may be emphasized in health education and physical education classes, many adults at the school may remain inactive. A mixed message about health and a lack of adult role modeling and support for health literacy can undermine the best health education program.

Components of a Coordinated School Health System

This chapter focuses on how schools can build a coordinated school health system to support and reinforce instruction on healthy behavior and health literacy. A coordinated school health system consists of eight components:

- Health Education
- Physical Education
- Health Services
- Nutrition Services
- Psychological and Counseling Services
- Health Promotion for Staff
- Safe and Healthy School Environment
- Parent and Community Involvement

Health Education

Health education, described in detail in Chapter 3, "Health Education," should be comprehensive and multidimensional and should not be limited to classroom exercises, textbook readings, or seat work. It should promote active student involvement, critical thinking, development and reinforcement of positive health behaviors, and a variety of engaging health-related projects both in and out of school. To complement the description of health education, the following discussion focuses on the other seven components of a coordinated school health system—how they are interrelated and how they can be supported and strengthened.

Physical Education

Physical education should provide all students with opportunities to participate in a comprehensive, sequentially planned physical education program. Through movement, physical education advances the physical, mental, emotional, and social well-being of every person in the pursuit of lifelong health. Students should have opportunities to develop and enhance their movement skills and their understanding of how their body moves and should participate in a variety of activities leading to lifelong enjoyment of physical activity. Physical education for children in kindergarten through grade twelve is the subject of another framework. Detailed information on the design of an effective physical education curriculum is provided in the *Physical Education Framework.*[1]

Health Services

Health services are those health-related procedures, screenings, or referrals coordinated at the school site by the credentialed school nurse or school-linked service providers. The nature and extent of health services vary from place to place. In general, however, all schools should be prepared to:

1. Treat minor illness and injuries, provide routine first aid, and assist in medical emergencies.
2. Identify and help manage the care of students with chronic conditions.
3. Conduct preventive health screenings, such as those for vision, hearing, or detection of scoliosis.
4. Refer the family to health providers in the community when problems are detected and do the necessary follow-up with the family as needed.
5. Keep up-to-date records of immunizations and health status.

Ten Benefits of Comprehensive School Health Systems

1. Less school vandalism
2. Improved attendance by students and staff
3. Reduced health care costs
4. Reduced substitute teaching costs
5. Better family communications, even on sensitive issues, such as sexuality
6. Stronger self-confidence and self-esteem
7. Noticeably fewer students using tobacco
8. Improved cholesterol levels for students and staff
9. Increased use of seat belts
10. Improved physical fitness

—*Healthy Kids for the Year 2000: An Action Plan for Schools*

---

[1] *Physical Education Framework for California Public Schools, Kindergarten Through Grade Twelve.* Sacramento: California Department of Education, 1994.

The school nurse is an invaluable asset to a coordinated school health system and represents a highly cost-effective community investment in the prevention of health problems.

An effective nutrition services program is basic to successful learning in schools. . . . Nutrition services can help to alleviate the physical signs and behaviors related to hunger and improve resistance to some communicable diseases.

According to the National Association of School Nurses, an acceptable nurse-to-student ratio is generally 1:750 but lower in schools with a concentration of special-needs students.[2] Most schools in California do not have a full-time nurse of their own. Often, a nurse or nurse practitioner spends time at two or more schools and may have to supervise one or more on-site health aides. This failure to provide adequate nursing is regrettable because the school nurse is an invaluable asset to a coordinated school health system and represents a highly cost-effective community investment in the prevention of health problems.

Another approach to providing health services and support to families can be found in the growing number of school-based or school-linked health services. These services may be offered by public health agencies or the school district and may be funded by a combination of public and private funds. In some communities school health clinics and school-linked services provide a range of health and support services, such as immunizations and acute care for infections, to students who might otherwise go without medical care and offer an excellent opportunity for school-community collaboration. The decision to provide school-linked support services and the guidelines for operating them are sensitive matters that should be determined by the local community and the school district governing board.

Nutrition Services

An effective nutrition services program is basic to successful learning in schools. Hungry children can neither learn nor achieve their potential in physical development, level of activity, or mental ability. Nutrition services can help to alleviate the physical signs and behaviors related to hunger and improve resistance to some communicable diseases. In addition, when received by pregnant teenagers, these services help to reduce the risk of developmental disabilities and greatly reduce infant mortality, a serious problem in teenage pregnancy. Depending on the needs of the students and the community, nutrition services might include breakfast and lunch programs, a summer feeding program, a pregnant and lactating teen program, a special milk program, and a child-care food program.

A national health goal is that at least 90 percent of the school lunch and breakfast programs provide food choices consistent with such dietary recommendations as those contained in *The California Daily Food Guide*.[3] Specifically, the goal is to increase the consumption of whole grains, fruits, and vegetables and moderate the consumption of fat, salt, sugar, and empty-calorie foods. In addressing this goal, nutrition services can offer students a variety of foods that promote optimal health while reflecting student preferences. However, the

[2] *Resolutions and Policy Statements.* Scarborough, Maine.: National Association of School Nurses, 1990, p. 22.

[3] *The California Daily Food Guide: Dietary Guidance for Californians.* Sacramento: California Department of Education, 1990.

school nutrition program does more than feed students; it functions as a living laboratory for the practice of good eating habits learned in the classroom. Nutrition services personnel can also be an invaluable resource to the classroom, providing assistance in nutrition-related lessons.

Psychological and Counseling Services

Psychological and counseling services at the school site provide students with support and assistance in making healthy decisions, managing emotions, coping with crises, and setting short-term and long-term goals. Symptoms of mental, emotional, and social problems may be especially apparent among adolescents, ranging from abuse of alcohol, tobacco, and other drugs to eating disorders, antisocial aggression, and suicidal depression. Early detection of mental and emotional problems among children in elementary school should also be an important priority. Further, psychological and counseling services can provide support to students and their families after disasters or violent occurrences at or near the school.

Every school should have a well-coordinated and fully supported program led by a certificated professional who can help identify students with high-risk behaviors and intervene early with necessary assistance to parents and referrals to appropriate agencies. The primary responsibility for these services should be assigned to a professional counselor whose time should not be monopolized by administrative duties. However, because student health is a schoolwide concern, every adult on campus should watch out for troubled youngsters and assist them in finding the help and support they need.

Health Promotion for Staff

Part of the value of a staff health-promotion program lies in the numerous personal benefits it can offer staff members. Consistent with the growing number of health and fitness programs supported by private industry, schools should view health promotion for staff as part of an overall approach to disease prevention and sound health policy. In addition, adults must view themselves as role models for healthy behavior if they are serious about helping young people achieve health literacy.

School-based health and fitness programs for staff members and other adults can take many forms, including work-site health promotion programs; health-risk appraisals; personal goal-setting sessions; support groups; employee assistance programs; and classes in aerobics, stress management, weight control, and smoking cessation. The common denominator throughout is teaching by example and promoting the health of all adults in the school.

Adults must view themselves as role models for healthy behavior if they are serious about helping young people achieve health literacy.

Safe and Healthy School Environment

This component relates to the physical and emotional environments of the school. Above all, a safe and healthy school environment ensures that the school is a haven from the violence many young people encounter elsewhere. Such an environment is one that is well maintained and is free of such hazards as asbestos dust or drinking water contaminated by lead. A plan to be implemented in case of fire or natural disasters or other emergencies should be provided and should be well rehearsed. In addition, lavatories and other sanitary facilities should be kept clean, supplied with soap and towels, and maintained well; play equipment should be inspected for safety at regular intervals; and the school grounds should be monitored and kept free of alcohol, tobacco, and other drugs.

The human side of a safe and healthy environment is less tangible but just as important. It involves effective leadership and a sense of collaboration and community. Healthy schools are characterized by a culture of concern and mutual support among staff members and students. The importance of social values—caring for others, treating others with respect, affirming diversity, and being a responsible member of a group—should be clearly stated, recognized, and modeled by all adults. Demeaning statements or actions directed to staff members or students should not be tolerated.

Parent and Community Involvement

Involving families and the community in the coordinated school health system is essential to encouraging positive health behaviors in children. Family values and community norms help shape the health decisions of young people. It follows, then, that if schools are to promote children's health literacy, they must reach out to key influence groups in the community. Working together, the school, the family, and the community can tailor the coordinated school health system to meet the school's specific needs.

Although the school receives support from family members in many different ways, it must uphold the role of the parent or guardian as the child's primary caretaker. To do so includes understanding and respecting the different ways in which families and cultural and ethnic groups may view health-related issues. It also includes a recognition that the law provides parents with basic rights regarding the review of certain health-related instructional materials and the option of removing their children from those parts of instructional programs dealing with health, family life education, or sex education that conflict with the parents' religious training or beliefs (*Education Code* Section 51513).

Interrelationships of Components

Each component of a coordinated school health system has its own characteristics and involves adults possessing distinct professional orientation and specialized skills. To view the components as completely independent and separate from each other is, however, inconsistent with the philosophy of a coordinated school health system and is counterproductive.

Taken together, all eight components make up a coordinated school health system. All relate to the development of health literacy in students, and all are important. The more school health planners can establish connections and interrelationships among the components, the stronger will be the overall coordinated school health system and the more positive will be the outcomes for children's health. A well-integrated system creates unity, coherence, and consistent support for students' health literacy. Rather than being limited to discrete time slots labeled *health,* the system permeates the school day. It is schoolwide, involving students and adults within the school and in the community.

The following discussion of connections and interrelationships focuses on two key aspects of organizing the coordinated school health system; that is, linkages within the school and linkages between the school and the community. Both are important to a successful coordinated school health system. Throughout, examples are used to illustrate ways in which interrelationships can be established and reinforced; however, they are not intended to constitute a complete or exhaustive list. Because there is no single correct way to organize a school health effort, specifics will vary from one setting to another.

A well-integrated school health system creates unity, coherence, and consistent support for students' health literacy.

Linkages Within the School

The most important principle for organizing and establishing relationships among the components of a coordinated school health system is the same as it is for health education; that is, interrelationships should be guided by the four unifying ideas of health literacy. All eight components should reinforce each other and complement the ways in which the unifying ideas are used to guide health education. Examples include the following:

Accepting Personal Responsibility

- The *physical education* program can emphasize the development of individual skills and talents and a positive attitude toward physical activity that contributes to lifelong health and fitness. Physical educators can encourage students to participate in physical activities and develop skills and talents involving movement and dance that can be used throughout their lives. By emphasizing children's abilities to meet physical challenges

Accepting personal
responsibility requires,
among other things, an
ability to gain access to
and use *health services*
when necessary or
appropriate.

and stay physically fit, physical education can help to enhance the relationship between acceptance of responsibility for one's physical well-being and consequent self-esteem.

- Accepting personal responsibility requires, among other things, an ability to gain access to and use *health services* when necessary or appropriate. The school nurse and school-linked health-care providers can play a role in reinforcing personal responsibility by encouraging students to learn more about the functioning of their bodies through periodic health screenings and treatment of minor injuries. Personal responsibility involves self-diagnostic skills—knowing, for example, whether and when it is important to see the school nurse or another health-care provider. Students who take regular medication will interact with the school nurse and may also need the assistance of the nurse from time to time.

- The *nutrition services* program can and should offer students a wide range of healthy food choices. Beyond choosing the food they eat, students can be encouraged to contribute to and design menus, focusing on healthy ingredients and varied methods of food preparation.

- *Health promotion for staff* can provide role modeling for students when the adults in the school demonstrate personal responsibility for their health and well-being. Joint staff-student games and physical activities can help to promote the idea that health and fitness are enjoyable pursuits for people of all ages.

Respecting and Promoting the Health of Others

- *Physical education* can reinforce respect for and promotion of the health of others by promoting an understanding of individual differences, effective teamwork, and cooperation. An important outgrowth of an effective physical education program is the development of positive, healthy relationships in children.

- Promotion of a *safe and healthy school environment* is particularly important in reinforcing respect for and promotion of others' health. The culture of the school should be one that values respect and caring for others and social and civic responsibility. One application of this culture of concern for others would be to make a safe and healthy school environment accessible to all. To do so, some schools may have to provide devices and facilities for those who are blind or deaf or are confined to wheelchairs.

- *Nutrition services* can encourage students to recognize the importance of healthy foods and menus for all students, promoting the importance of a schoolwide approach to nutrition that involves everyone. School nutrition policies can focus on a commitment to good health by calling for healthy food choices throughout the school—in the classroom and cafeteria and at sports events and extracurricular activities.

- *Parent and community involvement* can play a key role in fostering respect for and promotion of the health of others. When parents and community representatives are directly and frequently involved in the coordinated school health system, they are acknowledging the value and importance of school health efforts for all children. The school can and should reach out to parents and community members, encouraging them to be presenters, volunteers, helpers, planners, or participants in events and activities in and outside of the classroom. Workshops for parents or visits to the home by school-linked providers of services may help communicate the importance and attributes of a supportive home environment in which students have positive role models and nurturing families.

Understanding Growth and Development

- A key aspect of *physical education* is an understanding of the process of human growth and development, including ways in which a combination of proper diet and activity can contribute to lifelong health and prevention of disease. Also emphasized is the reality that people grow and develop at different rates yet in many ways are similar.
- *Psychological and counseling services* can help students and their families accept and understand numerous aspects of their own growth and development, including disabilities. Individual and group counseling can enhance students' self-esteem and minimize the self-doubt that often affects students in adolescence.
- *A safe and healthy school environment* acknowledges physical differences among students. For example, toilets, sinks, and drinking fountains are placed closer to the ground in areas used by younger students; all types of facilities are made accessible to those in wheelchairs; and emergency warning systems include a means of notifying deaf students and blind students.

Individual and group counseling can enhance students' self-esteem and minimize the self-doubt that often affects students in adolescence.

Using Health-Related Information, Products, and Services

- The school's *nutrition services* program can help prepare students to become well-informed consumers of healthy foods. The program can emphasize healthy foods in the daily menu and healthy food choices in the school cafeteria that extend to their ability to make well-informed decisions about food at home, in grocery stores and supermarkets, and in a variety of restaurants. It can also encourage students to be aware of the nutrient values of the foods they eat and information found on the labels of packaged foods.
- An awareness of health-related products, information, and services can be encouraged as part of the *safe and healthy school environment* component through efforts to inform students about aspects of the school environment

An important emphasis
in parent and community
involvement can be to make
students and their families
aware of community services
and resources available for
assistance in emergencies
and other health-care
and support needs.

that are health-promoting and those that need improvement. The school should use only nonpolluting, nontoxic chemicals and paints, for example, in cleaning and maintaining the physical plant. In many schools asbestos removal programs and other efforts to rid the environment of unhealthy chemicals or materials can be emphasized in health education. Less obvious environmental factors, such as building design, lighting, and sound deflection, can also be incorporated. Students can be involved in cleaning, maintaining, and enhancing the school building and grounds (for example, by planting trees and gardening) as one way of improving the school's physical plant and human climate.

- *Parent and community involvement* can play a critical role in making students aware of health-related resources in the community and of negative elements (for example, alcohol, tobacco, and other drugs or safety hazards) that might be a threat to children's health. An important emphasis in parent and community involvement can be to make students and their families aware of community services and resources available for assistance in emergencies and other health-care and support needs. Both formal resources (e.g., county agencies, community health-service providers) and informal resources (e.g., neighborhood groups, recreation clubs) should be featured.

- *Health promotion for staff* can and should encourage staff members themselves to be informed consumers of goods and services that can affect their health. Staff members can, in turn, share this knowledge with students, thereby enhancing their position as healthy role models and health-literate adults.

In addition to promoting the four unifying ideas of health literacy in students, the components of a coordinated school health system should be interrelated as much as possible. For example, specific organizing structures designed to advance health literacy schoolwide can be used. They may include frequent meetings of the school health committee and the coordinators of the eight components, such as teachers, nutrition services staff, nurses, school maintenance personnel, support staff, and parent and community volunteers. Another approach might be regular communication about the coordinated school health system within the school. Staff meetings can emphasize ways in which the components of the comprehensive health system complement and support each other. Bulletins, in-service events, and other communications can emphasize health-related activities. Events such as health fairs and health career days can further convey the priority of health at the school and the many different ways in which the school develops and supports health literacy.

Also important in linking the components and developing a unified, coherent approach to a coordinated school health system is continual emphasis on the conceptual and content linkages among the components. For example, all the components can support and relate to various aspects of *health education*.

Activities can be arranged and coordinated so that special events developed by *nutrition services* support the study of foods and nutrients in the classroom. And students' testing of respiratory rates and physical fitness in *physical education* can be coordinated with the study of human growth and development.

Involvement of the School, the Family, and the Community

A high degree of parent and community involvement is essential to unifying and strengthening the components of a coordinated school health system. Parent and community involvement should be encouraged from the earliest stages of program planning and conceptualization and should be cultivated as programs continue and expand.

Parents, other family members, and representatives of the community, including representatives of community agencies and organizations that provide health-related services, can be linked to the coordinated school health system in a variety of ways:

- Through emphasis on early identification of health problems, such as difficulties in seeing and hearing, recurrent infections, or chronic conditions, such as asthma, *health services* can promote parent and community involvement, underscoring the fact that everyone in the school and community has a role to play in maintaining the health of each child, no matter what the child's needs might be.

- In some cases students needing *psychological and counseling services* may have needs that cannot be met by the school's staff. Parents can then be referred to a variety of resources in the community.

- The *physical education* program can encourage students, their families, and staff members to take part in physical activity outside the school. Health clubs, sports leagues, programs sponsored by the local parks department or community-based organizations, family fun nights, organized hikes, and fund-raising walk-a-thons are all ways to show support and enthusiasm for vigorous physical activity.

- The *nutrition services* program can help strengthen school-community linkages by disseminating information broadly about the school's nutrition services and community food and nutrition programs. For example, monthly lunch and breakfast menus can be printed with nutrition-related news for parents and students, such as healthy, easy-to-prepare recipes; and periodic updates can be provided to the school board, relevant governmental agencies, and the local media. Working with local parent-teacher groups, school nutrition personnel can introduce food-related issues, such as the importance of a good breakfast in promoting academic performance or information on how nutrition habits at home and after

Working with local parent-teacher groups, school nutrition personnel can introduce food-related issues, such as the importance of a good breakfast in promoting academic performance or information on how nutrition habits at home and after school affect choices at school.

school affect choices at school. Good nutrition can also be promoted through collaboration with community groups and agencies, including professional associations interested in dietetics, medicine, child nutrition programs, and home economics and local community-based organizations that focus on youth and health issues. Connections with the food industry, including food producers, retail stores, and restaurants, are another way to promote the use of healthier food products throughout the community.

- The community can be involved in developing *health-promotion programs for school staff.* For example, local fitness centers may be able to offer group health-risk appraisals at reduced cost, and community health professionals can be invited to deliver informal noontime presentations on health to staff members.

- The community can also be involved in many different approaches to promoting a *safe and healthy school environment.* Above all, students should be encouraged to see the connections between all aspects of the environment, both in and out of school, and their own and others' health. Students should experience ways to give back to the community. For example, they can experience the satisfaction of helping others by visiting nursing homes, volunteering time at the local hospital, or collecting and distributing food for the homeless. Community service activities can be awarded credit toward graduation. Students can also be involved in community recycling programs. Students and teachers can organize ways to minimize air pollution from automobiles by coming to school in carpools or buses, on bicycles, or on foot. The school can communicate regularly about safety-related concerns with local emergency services agencies, law-enforcement agencies, fire-protection districts, and community-based organizations that can provide adults and students with training in such techniques as first aid and cardiopulmonary resuscitation.

Numerous other examples could be provided of effective ways to link the school, the family, and the community in health-related efforts. All can contribute to making the school and community an environment that promotes children's health. In addition, because in some cases the health of children can be improved only through direct services and support to families, the school-family-community linkages developed to support the coordinated school health system can be used to provide school-linked services and support to families when needed.

> Students should be encouraged to see the connections between all aspects of the environment, both in and out of school, and their own and others' health. Students should experience ways to give back to the community.

Local Advisory or Coordinating Councils

In recent years school health professionals have worked to create an infrastructure to support coordinated school health systems. Particularly important at a time of increasingly limited resources for school health is support at the local level. An approach that has proven successful is that of establishing a local school health council, sometimes called a school health advisory council.

Many different types of school health councils can be formed; there is no single established or accepted model and no specific mandate or type of funds for school health councils. Rather, the concept of school health councils has been advocated by several leadership organizations, most notably the American Cancer Society, and school districts are encouraged to develop school health councils that address their specific needs.

Primarily advisory in nature, school health councils are groups of persons who represent diverse segments of the community and who collectively advise the local school system on health-related issues, activities, and programs. Representatives might be community-based health professionals and volunteers, school nurses, health educators, school administrators, physical education teachers, parents, students, and others interested in and concerned about school health. As suggested by the American Cancer Society, a school health council may have several distinct but complementary functions, summarized as follows:

- **Program planning**—Organizing and participating in regular meetings to assess local needs and to address problems and concerns
- **Advocacy**—Promoting school health issues by giving them a priority in plans and the allocation of resources
- **Fiscal planning**—Assessing the financial needs of school health systems and identifying and integrating funding sources
- **Liaison with district and state agencies**—Working with the school district and local agencies to plan and develop curriculum and to allocate resources
- **Direct intervention**—Initiating policies and organizing health-related activities, such as school health fairs
- **Evaluation, accountability, and quality control**—Ensuring that funds and resources are being used effectively and assessing local needs on a continual basis[4]

To receive federal funds, such programs as Healthy Start and drug- and alcohol- prevention programs are often required to work collaboratively with similar agencies. When prevention programs collaborate, a broader base of

---

[4] *Improving School Health: A Guide to School Health Councils.* Developed by Christin P. Bellian. Atlanta: American Cancer Society, 1999.

health issues can be addressed effectively, and such collaboratives can qualify as local school health councils.

School health councils can be important to the Parent and Community Involvement component of a coordinated school health system. They can be useful in assessing community problems and identifying appropriate programs and solutions. As the California Center for Health Improvement (CCHI) noted in 2000, establishing a school health council not only allows communities to tailor health education programs to fit specific needs but also increases opportunities for family involvement.[5]

A successful example cited by CCHI is the Long Beach Unified School District's School Health Advisory Council, which began in 1992 as a drug, alcohol, and tobacco education advisory council as required by the Drug-Free Schools and Communities Act. In 1995 the council, which meets quarterly, expanded its focus to encompass all content areas of health education. Active council members include representatives of law enforcement agencies, city health departments, parent groups, student groups, the American Cancer Society, the American Heart Association, and the American Lung Association. Among the council's many functions is that of providing a forum for sharing information and connecting members from each of the eight components of a coordinated school health system. The council has also helped to review content standards for the district's health, HIV/AIDS, and family life curricula.[6] More information is available under "Health Policy Coach" at the CCHI Web site at <*http://www.cchi.org*>.

Health Services in Schools

Why should health services be a priority for California schools? Schools are ideal places in which to provide coordinated health and human services because most children older than five years of age attend school. Therefore, schools are logical places in which to provide such preventive health services as screenings for vision, hearing, scoliosis, and dental problems. California law requires not only that health screenings be provided (*Education Code* sections 49452 and 49452.5) but also that students be immunized against specific vaccine-preventable communicable diseases (*Health and Safety Code* Section 120335).

Schools bring together large numbers of students and staff. Reasonable caution requires that schools have an organized way of addressing all health issues, including first aid, chronic disease management, medical emergencies,

---

[5] "Involving the Family in School Health Advisory Councils." Policy profile prepared by the California Center for Health Improvement, Sacramento, 2000.

[6] "Family and Community Involvement: School Health Advisory Councils." Policy profile prepared by the California Center for Health Improvement, Sacramento, 2000.

the identification of communicable diseases, and child abuse identification and reporting. Schools must also provide for routine health care needs of students, such as the administration of medications (*Education Code* Section 49423). All these services require recordkeeping and management to ensure proper documentation and follow-up care.

The need for school health services has expanded significantly as the circumstances of both the schools and the health care systems have changed. Federal laws concerning special education students require that schools provide the services necessary for these students to receive an appropriate education. Examples of such services are the monitoring of vital signs, tracheostomy care and suctioning, dressing changes, catheterization, gastric tube feeding, and the administration of oxygen. Advances in medicine, reforms in federal law, and school reform movements have allowed many students with chronic health conditions, such as diabetes, cancer, arthritis, and severe asthma, to participate in regular education settings. Schools must have a system in place that allows for consultation with these students' families and physicians, and the system must be supervised by credentialed school nurses, who can also assist students with medications, special treatments, and equipment use. Schools must also provide health care services to students who develop acute health problems while at school.

Legislative mandates and necessary precautions related to risks and liability give schools little or no option in providing health services.[7] Schools must be prepared, for example, to deal with emergencies occurring on the school campus that require special procedures and appropriately trained staff. Such emergencies include severe allergic reactions; drug overdoses; choking; suicide attempts; student or teacher death; trauma related to violence; and serious unintentional injuries, such as playground and sports-related injuries.[8]

Many schools with adequate school nursing coverage, Healthy Start programs, or school-based or school-linked clinics offer health and social services that help resolve issues of access to health care and fill or reduce gaps in the community's health care system. School health personnel can provide information and counseling about safe and healthy lifestyle choices and risk reduction that may empower students to assume responsibility for their health and safety. Health counseling for students with health problems identified during treatment might address the use of tobacco, alcohol, and other drugs; HIV/AIDS and other bloodborne diseases; unintentional injuries; eating disorders or obesity; and other health-related problems that may affect a student's ability to learn.[9]

---

[7] *Schools and Health: Our Nation's Investment.* Edited by Diane Allensworth and others. Washington, D.C.: National Academy Press, 1997, p. 157.

[8] *Health Is Academic: A Guide to Coordinated School Health Programs.* Edited by Eva Marx, Susan Frelick Wooley, and Daphne Northrop. New York: Teachers College Press, 1998, p. 173.

[9] Ibid, pp. 174-75.

Options for Meeting Students' Health Services Needs

According to the American Academy of Pediatrics, as cited in *Schools and Health,* school health services should be viewed as a component of a communitywide health care system.[10] Using school health services for mandated screening and the identification of problems, follow-up, and referral can improve the accessibility, effectiveness, and efficiency of primary care. For students to benefit fully from health services, schools and communities need to work together. Every school should have a core of health services provided by credentialed school nurses and trained or licensed support personnel. The school and community, working in tandem, need to assess which additional health services schools will provide, considering students' health and educational needs and the availability of appropriate health services in the community.

Traditionally, credentialed school nurses are the backbone of school health services and are often the only health care professionals on the school campus. School nurses typically provide primary prevention and health care services in a school health office, with or without the assistance of a health aide. The National Association of School Nurses continues to recommend a ratio of one school nurse to no more than 750 students in regular education.[11]

Students with special needs who require specialized services may be served by school nurses as well as by licensed or nonlicensed assistive personnel; physical therapists; occupational therapists; braillists; orientation and mobility specialists; speech, language, and hearing therapists; and audiologists. The National Association of School Nurses recommends a ratio of one school nurse to no more than 125 special education students.[12]

Potential Funding Sources for School Health Services

Historically, school districts or individual schools have paid the cost of school health services out of district budgets. This practice has created an inconsistent funding base that has been a barrier to the establishment of universal school-based health services. In addition, student health and wellness have tended to remain a low priority and have not been recognized as having an impact on academic achievement. Consequently, no consensus exists within the educational establishment on the need for school health services when hard budget choices must be made. Therefore, it is important to look outside of school budgets for reliable sources of financial support for school health services.[13]

---

[10] *Schools and Health,* p. 217.

[11] *National Association of School Nurses Position Statement: Caseload Assignments.* National Association of School Nurses Web site *<http://208.5.177.157/positions/caseload.htm>*. 1995.

[12] Ibid.

[13] *Schools and Health,* p. 206.

Some federal funds are available for school health services. These funds include "entitlement" funds and reimbursement funds for services rendered. Fund sources include federal Title XIX, which in California is known as the Child Health and Disability Prevention program, and federal Titles I and V of the No Child Left Behind Act of 2001, which can provide funds for health care for educationally disadvantaged children. The Individuals with Disabilities Education Act is another potential fund source; it partially supports mandated specialized services for children with disabilities. Other federal resources include funds for services to prevent HIV/AIDS and hepatitis B, funds for services to prevent drug use through the Safe and Drug Free Schools and Communities Act (Title IV), and the model coordinated school health programs of the U.S. Department of Education (which may include health services).

Through the Mandated Cost Program, districts may file claims with the State Controller's Office to be reimbursed for mandated scoliosis screening and related follow-up activities and for time spent auditing and following up on immunization and first-grade physical examination requirements. In addition, California has provided funds to support tobacco-use prevention and health care for children and families living in poverty. Healthy Start grants fund a variety of health and social services for eligible schools. In California the Local Educational Agency Medi-Cal Billing Option, which allows school districts to bill for health-related services provided to eligible students by appropriately licensed employees, has generated millions of dollars statewide for participating districts.

Local service clubs, volunteer health organizations (such as the American Lung Association, the American Cancer Society, the American Heart Association, and the American Red Cross), and private providers in the community may provide funds or in-kind contributions for a school health services program. Managed care organizations are increasingly willing to work with schools to provide health care services at school for students who are members of their plan or to develop school-linked clinics for such care.

Although California's Healthy Families and Medi-Cal for Children programs do not provide direct funds to schools, hundreds of children have the opportunity to obtain low-cost or free health care coverage through participation in these programs. Schools are in a unique position to help ensure that students and families have access to these and other affordable health coverage programs. Healthy Families and Medi-Cal for Children offer comprehensive medical, dental, and vision care coverage for children from low- to moderate-income families. Benefits are well-child care, immunizations, prescription medicine, dental and vision care (including prescription eyeglasses), mental health services, and physician and hospital services.

The following examples illustrate some of the student health problems that significantly affect schools:

- Nearly one in 13 school-age children has asthma. Asthma is a leading cause of school absenteeism, accounting for more than ten million absences per school year.[14]
- The number of children with diabetes has increased dramatically in recent years, requiring school personnel to be educated in ways to recognize emergency signs and symptoms and to intervene when necessary.[15]
- Oral disease is the most common childhood health problem. Children in California have twice the rate of untreated tooth decay as do their national counterparts.[16]

The volume and complexity of the need for health services for students are indeed challenging for schools. It is imperative that schools establish policies and protocols to manage those health-services needs. Qualified staff must be in place and trained in protocols and procedures for the protection of students, staff, and the school.

As noted in *Schools and Health: Our Nation's Investment,* the American Academy of Pediatrics has established the following seven guidelines for establishing school health programs:

1. Ensure access to primary health care.
2. Provide a system for dealing with crisis medical situations.
3. Provide mandated screening and immunization monitoring.
4. Provide systems for identification and solution of students' health and education problems.
5. Provide comprehensive and appropriate health education.
6. Provide a healthful and safe school environment that facilitates learning.
7. Provide a system of evaluation of the effectiveness of the school health program.[17]

Mental Health Issues in Schools

Mental health is one aspect of students' health and well-being that many educators tend to overlook. Yet mental health is an essential factor in students' attitude toward themselves and in their ability to succeed in a variety of settings, both in and out of school. Educators may be uncomfortable in dealing

---

[14] *Managing Asthma in the School Environment.* Washington, D.C.: U.S. Environmental Protection Agency, 2000.

[15] "American Diabetes Association Position Statement: Care of Children with Diabetes in the School and Day Care Setting," *Diabetes Care,* Vol. 25 (2002), S122-26.

[16] Mary Vaiana and Ian Coulter, *The Oral Health of California's Children: Halting the Neglected Epidemic—California Children's Dental Health Initiative.* Oakland, Calif.: The Dental Health Foundation, 2000.

[17] *Schools and Health,* p. 217.

with this aspect of young people's development because of the challenge of addressing mental health effectively and appropriately. Although teachers are often the first adults to see that a student may be experiencing emotional distress, teachers do not have the professional knowledge or expertise to diagnose or treat mental health problems. Ignoring a student's mental health needs, however, is not an option. Schools and districts should develop referral policies and procedures for dealing with mental health issues, and the procedures need to be communicated clearly through sufficient staff training.

Psychological and counseling services are one of the eight components of a coordinated school health system. This component holds an important place in a well-designed school health program because a pressing need for it exists. Howard Adelman notes that "between 12 percent and 22 percent of all children suffer from a diagnosable mental, emotional, or behavioral disorder, and relatively few receive mental health services."[18] According to Adelman, "Counseling, psychological and social services are essential for youngsters experiencing severe and pervasive problems."[19] He states that these problems include the following:

- *Inadequate basic resources,* such as food, clothing, housing, and a sense of security at home, school, and in the neighborhood
- *Psychosocial problems,* such as difficult relationships at home and at school; emotional upsets; language problems; sexual, emotional, or physical abuse; substance abuse; delinquent or gang-related behavior; psychopathology
- *Stressful situations,* such as being unable to meet the demands made at school or at home, inadequate support systems, and hostile conditions at school or in the neighborhood
- *Crises and emergencies,* such as the death of a classmate or relative, a shooting at school, or natural disasters (e.g., earthquakes, floods, tornadoes)
- *Life transitions,* such as the onset of puberty, a move to a new school, and changes in life or family circumstances (e.g., change of residence, immigration, loss of a parent through divorce or death)[20]

Seen in this light, the mental health needs and challenges of students take on a more recognizable and everyday nature. A key question, then, is How can schools work with families and community supports to address mental health needs appropriately and effectively? Several statutes specify the referral procedures for mental health concerns, and more detail on those statutes can be

---

[18] Howard Adelman, "School Counseling, Psychological, and Social Services," in *Health Is Academic: A Guide to Coordinated School Health Programs.* Edited by E. Marx, S. F. Wooley, and D. Northrop. New York: Teachers College Press, 1998, p. 142.

[19] Ibid., p. 143.

[20] Ibid.

found in Chapter 2, "Developing Health Literacy in the Classroom and in the School." The protection of education rights for students with disabilities is guaranteed by the following legislation:

1. The federal Individuals with Disabilities Education Act (IDEA) (20 *United States Code [USC]* sections 1400 et seq.; and 34 *Code of Federal Regulations [CFR],* parts 300 and 303)
2. The federal Rehabilitation Act, Section 504 (29 *USC* 705 [20] and 794; and 34 *CFR,* Part 104)
3. The federal Americans with Disabilities Act (ADA) (42 *USC* 12101–12213; 47 *USC* 225, 611; and 28 *CFR,* Part 35)
4. *Education Code,* Part 30 (sections 56000 et seq.)
5. *California Code of Regulations, Title 5* (sections 3000 et seq.)
6. *Government Code,* Chapter 26.5 (sections 7570 et seq.) of Division 7 of Title 1

More information on the education rights of students with disabilities is available at the Web site *<http://www.cde.ca.gov/spbranch/sed/lawsreg2.htm>.*

Although not specifically identified in Chapter 3, "Health Education," as being a part of a distinct mental health category, numerous themes that are closely associated with mental health are woven throughout the description of the health curriculum in that chapter. These themes cover the following topics:

- Mental and emotional health
- Growth and development
- Alcohol, tobacco, and other drugs
- Child abuse, including sexual exploitation
- Roles of family members
- Change within the family
- Friendship and peer relationships
- Sexuality

Adelman recommends using school-based strategies for prevention, intervention, and treatment.[21] After a professional assessment of students' needs is made, the services of school personnel—such as counselors, psychologists, social workers, and nurses—should be implemented. Links between school and community programs and services should be established to provide students with the appropriate resources, opportunities, skills development, and formal instruction supports they need.

All programs and services should be supported by policies and appropriate training for staff to recognize the triggers for referring students for a professional assessment of their needs. The policies must be in compliance with IDEA. A checklist of IDEA criteria is available at the CDE Web site at *<http://www.cde.ca.gov/spbranch/sed>.*

---

[21] Ibid.

The California Public Mental Health System and Schools

California has a decentralized public mental health service delivery system, and most services for adults and children are provided through the county mental health departments. Many communities have multiple providers of mental health services. Most insurers, health maintenance organizations, and public insurance providers, such as Healthy Families, offer coverage for mental health services. The public mental health system is intended to provide a safety net for persons who have no other mental health care resources.

County mental health professionals can be contacted primarily by school psychologists or nurses participating in the individualized education programs. These health professionals can be valuable assets to school health councils and multidisciplinary school health teams. They can help set up systems for student referrals and provide mental health expertise.

In addition, the local mental health department is responsible for the administration and delivery of several publicly funded services for children and youths. Collaboration between schools and the public mental health system provides an opportunity to maximize cost effectiveness and to meet students' needs that can interfere with academic success if they go unmet.

Services available to children through California's public mental health system are as follows:

Medi-Cal

Medi-Cal (California's name for the federal Medicaid program) is a health insurance program that provides medical assistance for low-income persons. It is funded through a state and federal partnership. Federal statutes require states to provide diagnostic and treatment services to Medicaid recipients under the age of twenty-one regardless of whether the state provides the same benefits under its state Medicaid plan. In response, California has expanded its services to include the Early Periodic Screening, Diagnosis, and Treatment program. Funds can also be used to provide substance-abuse services to children with simultaneous mental illness and substance-abuse diagnoses when necessary to ameliorate the mental health problems of the child.

The Medi-Cal mental health care benefit is the most important part of community-based services that are available to low-income students and families. This benefit is a significant resource for school professionals to keep in mind as they seek support for families of students who have been identified, formally or informally, as having behavioral or emotional difficulties.

The public mental health system generally delivers the following community-based and hospital-based Medi-Cal services through a network of the state's 58 counties:

- Crisis services
- Comprehensive evaluation and assessment
- Individual, family, and group services
- Medication education and management
- Case management
- Therapeutic behavioral services
- Habilitative and intensive day treatment
- Residential services (hospital)
- Hospital in-patient services

These services are provided or arranged by the local mental health departments.

Special Education Program

Legislation provides for the combining of educational and mental health resources in an interagency delivery model to offer, in conjunction with the educational system, specialty mental health services to students (*Government Code* sections 7570–88). These federally mandated services are an important entitlement for students who need the specific support of mental health services to achieve academic success. This interagency program designates the county mental health programs as the entities responsible for providing mental health services to students who require special education, who have been determined to be in need of mental health treatment in order to benefit from their education, and who have exhausted all regular school counseling services and still need additional counseling. The referral process and assessment process are very stringent, and the policies must be clearly defined and communicated to staff.

Children's System of Care

Another program of the state Department of Mental Health is the Children's System of Care (CSOC). In 1987 legislation was enacted that encouraged the development of organized, community-based CSOCs for emotionally disturbed (ED) children. The success of a planning model developed in Ventura County led to the state requiring the following core values for a CSOC: (1) the target population is composed of children and youths identified as ED; (2) the services are culturally competent and child- and family-centered; (3) the families are an integral part of the service planning and delivery; and (4) the children are, whenever possible, served at home or in the most home-like setting possible. Because the system recognizes that many children receive services from more than one agency (e.g., juvenile justice, education, social services, child welfare, and mental health), services should involve formal collaboration and coordination among the agencies. Typically, CSOC activities are coordinated with special student study teams on campus or with school attendance review boards working to meet the needs of students who have intense emotional or behavioral needs.

Early Mental Health Initiative

The Early Mental Health Initiative (EMHI) is a part of the continuum of mental health services administered by the state Department of Mental Health. A preventive service for children, EMHI was established to fund three-year demonstration programs serving school-aged children in kindergarten through grade three who are identified as having moderate adjustment problems at school. The purpose of EMHI is to ensure that these children start out well in school and to increase the likelihood of their success in school.

Safe Schools and Violence Prevention

Ensuring a safe and healthy learning environment in which conflict is effectively managed and minimized requires the collaborative efforts of all school staff. Creating a safe school environment also requires the involvement of parents and community partners, such as law enforcement and mental health service providers. School psychologists, counselors, nurses, social workers, child welfare and attendance supervisors, community partners, and others involved in student support services must work as a team to assess students' needs. This team must also assist teachers and parents with programs and services that support academic achievement and healthy development for all students.

The Safe and Healthy Kids Program Office (SHKPO) of the California Department of Education provides assistance to county offices of education, school districts, and schools through programs that address school safety. The School/Law Enforcement Partnership (S/LEP), which is managed jointly by SHKPO and the Attorney General's Crime and Violence Prevention Center, provides information, publications, conferences, and technical assistance on school safety through the services of its members—a group of professionals from law enforcement, education, and youth-serving agencies.

Education Code Section 35294 directs kindergarten-through-grade-twelve public schools to develop a comprehensive school safety plan by coordinating with school personnel, parents, students, and local law enforcement representatives to develop site-based safe school plans. These plans must (1) identify comprehensive approaches to school, student, and staff safety; (2) demonstrate the ways in which the school's vision incorporates school safety; (3) include an assessment of recent incidents of school crime, areas of desired change, and expected measurable outcomes; and (4) demonstrate a collaboratively designed action plan for implementing site-appropriate safety programs and strategies, including the expected fiscal impact of executing them. Schools are to integrate their safe school plan with other school improvement activities to prevent or reduce violence and to provide or maintain a high level of safety conducive to learning. Detailed information on the S/LEP program can be viewed at the SHKPO Web site at *<http://www.cde.ca.gov/healthykids>* or at the Crime and Violence Prevention Center Web site at *<http://caag.state.ca.us/cvpc>*.

The connection between problem solving and partnering is the focus of the School Community Policing Partnership Program. This program offers an opportunity for educational agencies and policing agencies to analyze problems and develop solutions through innovative and collaborative thinking. *Education Code* Section 32296.3 defines *school community policing* as an approach to safe schools in which schools, law enforcement, community agencies, and the members of the surrounding school community collaboratively develop long-term solutions to address the underlying conditions that affect the level of school safety. Detailed information is available from the School-Community Policy Partnership Program, telephone (916) 445-5629 or the Web site at *<http://www.cde.ca.gov/spbranch/ssp>*, or the Crime and Violence Prevention Center Web site at *<http://caag.state.ca.us/cvpc>*.

The Carl Washington School Safety and Violence Prevention Act provides entitlements for school safety on the basis of student enrollments in grades eight through twelve to school districts and county offices of education. Funds can be used for such strategies as hiring personnel trained in conflict resolution, providing on-campus communication devices, establishing staff training programs, and establishing cooperative arrangements with law enforcement. More information is available from SHKPO, telephone (916) 319-0920.

School Crime Information

Another responsibility of the SHKPO is the collection of data on the type and frequency of crime in schools to provide the Legislature and the California Department of Education with the necessary information to "permit development of effective programs and techniques to combat crime on school campuses" (*Penal Code* sections 628 et seq.). Historically, the collection of these data has been accomplished through the California Safe Schools Assessment (CSSA), a statewide uniform process for collecting school crime data at all school sites. As additions to the *Health Framework* were being written, CSSA was in abeyance while new data collection systems were being designed to meet the requirements of the federal No Child Left Behind (NCLB) Act and the California Budget Act of 2003.

According to Section 4112 of Title IV.A of NCLB, these new systems must collect data from each kindergarten-through-grade-twelve public school in California to provide information on truancy and suspensions and on expulsions for violent or drug-related offenses. Each district must provide information on the types of prevention programs and curricula being used in the district and data on the prevalence of and attitudes toward drug use and violence among youths.

In addition, Section 9532 of Title IX of NCLB requires the California Department of Education, in consultation with local educational agencies, to identify "persistently dangerous" schools. Such identification will require the collection of data on the most serious offenses committed at schools, most likely through the use of a subset of the data described above. A report to the Legislature in March 2003 contained details of the proposed systems outlined for meeting these federal requirements.

Threat Assessment

Threat assessment is a complex concept; the delineation of one threat from another depends on the person involved in making the threat, the threat itself, and the intended victim or victims of the threat. Because each situation is unique, threat assessment should be viewed as a process in which each case is handled very carefully and assessment is made in relation to the specific case, not generalized with other cases. Profiling (the use of behavioral or demographic characteristics to identify types of persons likely to become violent) and the use of checklists or other standardized assessment instruments have not proven to be effective in assessing individual cases.[22] Further, when used inappropriately, these techniques may result in stereotyping and inappropriate action.

Education Code sections 48900 et seq. address the issue of violence, including threats, and outline the grounds for suspension and expulsion. Specifically, Section 48900 authorizes suspension or a recommendation for expulsion of any student who has "caused, attempted to cause, or threatened to cause physical injury to another person. . . . " Behavior that qualifies for sanction is defined as "sufficiently severe or pervasive to have the actual and reasonably expected effect of materially disrupting classwork, creating substantial disorder, and invading the rights of either school personnel or pupils by creating an intimidating or hostile educational environment" (Section 48900.4).

The *Education Code* further authorizes suspension or a recommendation for expulsion when a student engages in sexual harassment; hate violence; harassment, threats, or intimidation; or terrorist threats against school officials, school property, or both (as defined in sections 48900.2–48900.4, 48900.7). A "terroristic threat" is defined as " . . . any statement, whether written or oral, by a person who willfully threatens to commit a crime which will result in death, great bodily injury to another person, or property damage in excess of one thousand dollars ($1,000), with the specific intent that the statement is to

---

[22] M. Reddy and others, "Evaluating Risk for Targeted Violence in Schools: Comparing Risk Assessment, Threat Assessment, and Other Approaches," *Psychology in the Schools,* Vol. 38, No. 2 (2001), 157–72.

be taken as a threat, even if there is no intent of actually carrying it out, which, on its face and under the circumstances in which it is made, is so unequivocal, unconditional, immediate, and specific as to convey to the person threatened, a gravity of purpose and an immediate prospect of execution of the threat, and thereby causes that person reasonably to be in sustained fear for his or her own safety or for his or her immediate family's safety, or for the protection of school district property, or the personal property of the person threatened or his or her immediate family" (Section 48900.7).

Violence Prevention and Targeted Threat Assessment Process

A violence prevention and targeted threat assessment process consists of three important elements:

1. A clearly understood system for safe and confidential reporting of threats
2. Ongoing staff development
3. A preventive assessment process

The first element is a *safe and confidential reporting system* that is known and understood by all students and developed by the school to meet its unique needs. Students should be educated on the importance of reporting threats of violence to the proper school authorities and of understanding that remaining silent can be dangerous to themselves as well as to others. Violence prevention training for students may cover interpersonal communication, conflict resolution, anger management, recognition of signs of depression, ways of coping with family tensions, and identification and reporting of threatening behavior.[23] Means of encouraging students to report threats of violence include the installation of a telephone line for anonymous tips or a drop-box with forms for reporting tips; the training and designation of selected adults as "safe contacts"; and the establishment of a "safe room" monitored by a trained adult.

The second element is an *ongoing staff development program* that prepares all staff to work together to develop a safe campus. Staff development programs should be chosen carefully to meet the needs of the school-site staff and should include training in targeted threat assessment and the social and emotional development of students. Specialized training is needed for those persons assigned to conduct or supervise the targeted threat assessment process. A needs assessment of the school climate is conducted to determine at which point on the learning continuum (awareness, knowledge, or skills) the staff development should begin. The county office of education, the local department of mental health, the California Department of Education, the Attorney General's Office, or the local law enforcement agency may be contacted for professional development training. Topics for training may include safe-schools planning, classroom

---

[23] Mary Ellen O'Toole, *The School Shooter: A Threat Assessment Perspective.* Quantico, Va.: Federal Bureau of Investigation, 2000.

management, crisis prevention and response, and appropriate responses to hate-motivated behavior.

The third element is a *preventive assessment process* to identify students who have the potential for violence. There is no common profile or set of characteristics that applies to the perpetrator of targeted violence; therefore, "violence is seen as the product of an interaction among the perpetrator, situation, target, and the setting."[24] It is very difficult to distinguish between the making of a threat and the posing of a threat. Relying solely on zero tolerance policies has not always proved to be effective and can create legal entanglements for schools and school districts. The following process is recommended for working with students who may pose a threat:

1. Interview the individual student. Try to determine whether the student is hostile or depressed, whether a desire to harm self or others exists, and whether the student has made a specific plan and logistical preparations to carry out the plan.

2. Corroborate the findings of the interview with cumulative behavioral, emotional, and academic records. Check the records to determine whether the student has any history of school problems, has family problems, experiences isolation, or has a history of having been socially excluded or bullied by peers.

3. Check with the adults, teachers, parents, and community members who interact daily with the student. Interview these adults to determine whether threats have been made, a plan has been revealed, the student's behavior has recently changed, or the student has had a recent loss or traumatic experience. An intervention team of student support services personnel should be available to assist in this process.

4. Elicit the help of skilled professionals to determine whether the findings warrant further investigation or reporting. Consult with the school counselor, school psychologist, or other mental health professional and develop a plan of involvement and support for the student.

5. Report to school officials and law enforcement authorities if there is suspicion of a threat or a threat has been made. A procedure for investigating threats should be developed collaboratively by schools and law enforcement agencies.

A targeted threat does not appear in isolation and usually involves more than one member of the school community; therefore, effective threat assessment and prevention must be a community or collaborative effort. School officials, student support services and mental health personnel, faculty and staff, parents, and law enforcement personnel must collaborate to develop and implement strategies that prevent threats and violence. Multidisciplinary school site teams

---

[24] M. Reddy and others, "Evaluating Risk," p. 167.

should be used to identify strategies and resources to help individual students and support schoolwide violence-prevention programs. In addition to the threat assessment process, prevention programs may include the use of volunteer mentors, parent volunteers, peer counselors, school counselors, and school resource officers. Other preventive strategies include arranging for public service announcements encouraging students to report disturbing behavior or threats, setting up peer assistance groups, educating parents on recognizing possible early warning signs in their children and obtaining help for them, organizing student assistance programs, and arranging "lunch buddy" programs in which approved adults interact with students.

Suicide Prevention

A more subtle type of violence is harm to oneself, which takes various forms that include eating disorders and suicide. The National Strategy for Suicide Prevention (NSSP), a collaborative effort of the Substance Abuse and Mental Health Services Administration, Centers for Disease Control and Prevention, National Institutes of Health, and Health Resources and Services Administration, has noted that suicide is the third leading cause of death for people between fifteen and twenty-four years of age. It is the fourth leading cause of death in children between ten and fourteen years of age. Although suicide attempts are more frequent among females, males are four times more likely to die from suicide attempts.[25]

The percentage of young suicide victims who tell someone of their plans beforehand is widely disputed among specialists in the field of adolescent suicide. However, the general agreement is that many young people do alert someone of their plan to take their own life. Research from the American Association of Suicidology shows that students are more likely to to tell another child closer to their own age than they are tell an adult.[26] Therefore, teachers and other educators need to watch for prolonged periods of moodiness or depression in their students.

When teachers have a concern about a student or receive information that may cause concern, they should consult with experienced student support personnel (e.g., school counselors, school psychologists, school social workers, or school nurses) or community mental health specialists, or both, to determine students' risk factors and the need for counseling. Students should be encouraged to tell their parents, teachers, administrators, counselors, and other student support personnel if they are, or someone they know is, having thoughts of suicide.

---

[25] *National Strategy for Suicide Prevention: Goals and Objectives for Action.* Washington, D.C.: U.S. Department of Health and Human Services, 2001.

[26] *Guidelines for School-Based Suicide Prevention Programs.* Washington, D.C.: American Association of Suicidology, 1999.

An analysis by the U.S. Department of Health and Human Services suggests that strategies can be grouped into two areas: strategies for enhancing the identification and referral of students at risk of suicide and strategies for addressing risk factors directly. Education for school personnel in both of these areas is essential because suicide-prevention programs included in the health curriculum have met with mixed results.

The following goals and objectives have been proposed by NSSP to enhance the identification and referral of students at risk of suicide and to address the risk factors directly:

1. Promote awareness that suicide is a public health problem that is preventable.
2. Adopt broad-based support for suicide prevention.
3. Adopt strategies to reduce the stigma associated with being a consumer of services related to mental health, substance abuse, and suicide prevention.
4. Adopt suicide prevention programs.
5. Promote efforts to reduce access to lethal means and methods of self-harm.
6. Implement training for recognition of at-risk behavior and delivery of effective treatment.
7. Adopt effective clinical and professional practices.
8. Improve access to and community linkages with mental health services and substance-abuse services.
9. Improve reports and portrayals of suicidal behavior, mental illness, and substance abuse in the entertainment and news media.
10. Promote and support research on suicide prevention.[27]

The implementation of these goals and objectives requires that school staff be trained in the identification and referral of students at risk of suicide and in strategies for addressing risk factors directly. Such training should be included in district staff development training plans.

The School Health Ship

An appropriate metaphor for the entire process of planning and implementing a coordinated school health system is the analogy of building a ship and setting sail, as illustrated in figures 2 and 3.

Essential to the ship's stability is health education. The ship's keel and ribs, which support the sheathing of the hull, are the nine different content areas. The four unifying ideas of health literacy connect the content areas and, with the content areas, form the hull.

---

[27] *National Strategy for Suicide Prevention.*

However, health education and health-related information are only one element of a total approach to developing health literacy in children and youths.

The ship's sails, which catch the energy of motivation, direction, and purpose in the lives of individuals, institutions, and communities, are the seven other components of a coordinated school health system.

Finally, the individual child, and ultimately every adult, is the captain of the ship, steering it in the direction of a healthy, successful life.

Fig. 2. Building the Hull of the Ship (Knowledge, Attitudes, Behaviors)

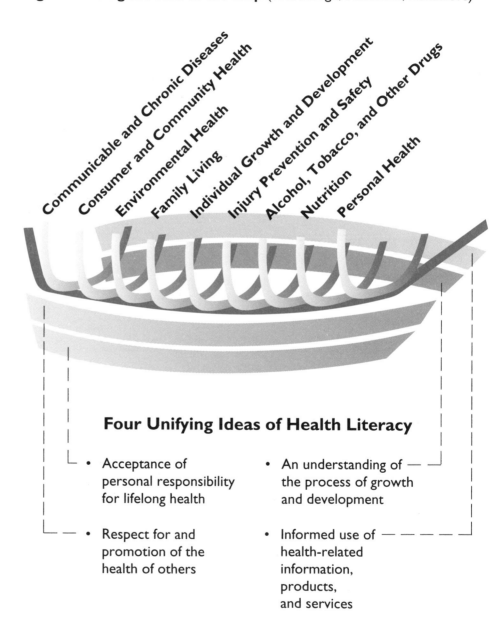

Four Unifying Ideas of Health Literacy

- Acceptance of personal responsibility for lifelong health

- Respect for and promotion of the health of others

- An understanding of the process of growth and development

- Informed use of health-related information, products, and services

All those who plan and carry out components of the coordinated school health system—in the school and in the community, as professionals, family members, or volunteers—can help to build a sound and sturdy ship for today's children and youths. When the ship is well designed and well constructed, it will be ready to weather the storms of life and take advantage of the gentle breezes that make life fulfilling.

Fig. 3. Set Your Sails (Harnessing the Energy)

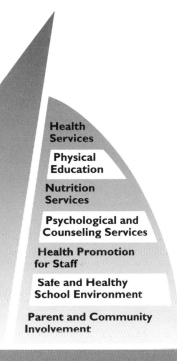

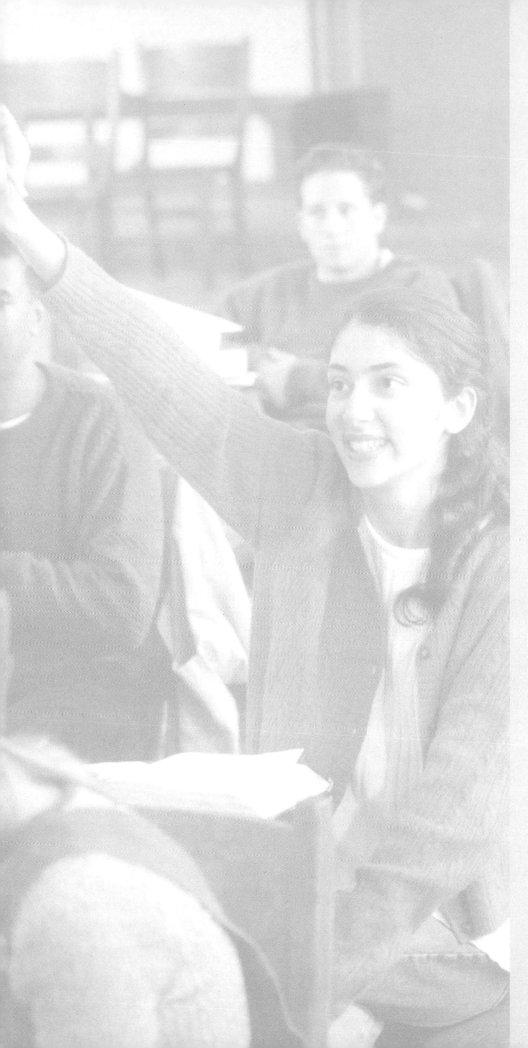

CHAPTER 5

Assessment
of Health
Literacy

Assessment approaches aligned with the desired expectations described in this framework are pivotal to the promotion of health literacy in children and youths. Since it is true that what is tested strongly influences what is taught, meaningful assessment focused on the knowledge, skills, attitudes, and behaviors necessary for health literacy should be built into curriculum design and the supporting structure from the outset.

Appropriate assessment will focus on the unifying ideas of health literacy. That is, it will attempt to measure students' progress toward:

- Accepting personal responsibility for lifelong health
- Respecting and promoting the health of others
- Understanding the process of growth and development
- Becoming informed users of health-related information, products, and services

The primary purpose of assessment should be to provide meaningful feedback to the student and teacher so that individual growth can be noted and future learning can be tailored to the student's needs. However, assessments in health education should be constructed to serve other important purposes. Because the health of students is influenced by the family, the community, the school, and peers, assessments should be designed to provide feedback to these groups. That is, assessment results should help parents, the community, and the students themselves understand the progress made toward health literacy for all students. These groups can use assessment results to help focus their efforts to support the development of health literacy and track progress over time.

Assessments also can provide valuable information for focusing and planning improvements in the coordinated school health system.[1] Because student health literacy is best achieved when health education is provided within the context of a coordinated school health system, effective assessment of health literacy must go beyond collecting only student-level data. Assessment should also examine the extent to which staff and the coordinated school health system promote and reinforce health literacy. Such assessment results, together with data from student assessments, can provide the information necessary to plan improvements in the coordinated school health system. When implemented, these improvements can further promote the development of health literacy in all students. Assessments should:

- Be consistent with the unifying ideas of this framework.
- Focus on knowledge, skills, attitudes, and behaviors rather than on knowledge only.
- Provide useful feedback to individual students, teachers, and parents.
- Include the gathering of baseline health literacy data so that behavioral change can be tracked over time.

> The primary purpose of assessment should be to provide meaningful feedback to the student and teacher so that individual growth can be noted and future learning can be tailored to the student's needs.

> Assessments should measure the extent to which the coordinated school health system enhances and reinforces health literacy.

[1] See Chapter 1 for an explanation of the coordinated school health system.

- Measure the extent to which the coordinated school health system enhances and reinforces health literacy.
- Promote ongoing refinement of both health education and the entire coordinated school health system.

Student Assessment

In the planning of student assessment in health, the following principles underlying effective assessment should be considered and integrated into the assessment design:

- The assessment should examine the extent to which all students are achieving the four unifying ideas of health literacy.
- Rather than measuring knowledge only, the assessment should focus on health knowledge, healthy behaviors, attitudes about health, and skills to increase the prevalence of positive health behaviors and reduce the prevalence of negative health behaviors.
- The assessment should revolve around exemplary tasks aligned with this framework that provide information about student performance.
- The assessment tasks should be complex, open-ended, and meaningful. They should allow students to demonstrate thinking, understanding, and communication skills as well as mastery of health content. In contrast to traditional assessments, they should provide sufficient flexibility in approach so that students have opportunities to demonstrate health literacy in a variety of ways. An understanding should prevail that a variety of ways to solve a problem correctly may exist. Students should have ample time to work on assessment tasks and opportunities to revise and resubmit projects to raise performance to high-quality standards.
- Whenever possible, the assessment should be conducted in the course of normal work. The class and the learning should not, in most cases, be interrupted for a test.
- The primary purpose of the assessment should be to provide meaningful feedback to the student, parents, and teacher so that future learning can be tailored to the student's needs and parents can understand and support this learning.

Assessments based on these principles will include much more than the traditional methods of assessment, such as multiple choice, true-false, or machine-scored measures of acquired knowledge. A wide array of assessment methods and instruments that measure behavior and skill development and support critical thinking and a student-centered curriculum should be used to assess student health literacy. Examples of student assessments include:

- Using self-assessments that include a risk assessment or personal inventory to give students an understanding of their health status

A wide array of
assessment methods
and instruments which
measure behavior and
skill development and
support critical thinking
and a student-centered
curriculum should be
used to assess student
health literacy.

- Using the results of a health-related physical fitness test to evaluate students' fitness level and to develop a personal fitness plan based on their level of fitness, knowledge acquired, and personal needs[2]
- Demonstrating an understanding of the connection between current behaviors and lifelong health by developing realistic and long-term goals related to health
- Role-playing ways to respond to physical, emotional, mental, and social changes that occur in a lifetime, including identifying available resources if needed
- Using positive social skills in small-group and large-group assignments with other students to work effectively toward a common goal
- Demonstrating specific decision-making, refusal, and conflict-resolution skills when given sample scenarios that allow students to grapple, in a safe environment, with difficult situations likely to happen during their lifetimes
- Reflecting, in journal entries, on the skills learned in the classroom and the use of those skills in the classroom, at school, with friends, or at home and indicating how those skills influence attitudes and behavior
- Recording food consumption in food diaries and using the diaries to analyze eating habits
- Developing a set of criteria for making decisions about health products that allow students to demonstrate an understanding of how marketing influences decision making
- Developing and using anonymous schoolwide surveys to obtain and analyze group data regarding negative and positive health behaviors, giving an important overall picture of the behavioral trends of students over time
- Developing and using student materials for schoolwide use that encourage actions and behaviors promoting good health, such as videos offering tips on skateboard, bicycle, and personal safety or a laminated poster illustrating emergency escape routes for each classroom
- Developing student portfolios that demonstrate the student's health literacy by addressing each of the four unifying ideas

One of the most effective ways to assess student progress toward health literacy is to observe whether their behavior supports or improves their health. However, before assessments of behaviors are focused on, two cautionary notes are in order. First, what a student learns in health education may not produce observable behavioral changes until much later. To expect immediate change is unrealistic. Second, assessment of behavior must be carefully constructed to respect students' rights to privacy, community sensibilities, and existing laws and notification requirements. *Education Code* Section 51513 requires parental permission to ask questions about the students' personal beliefs or practices and the parents' or guardians' beliefs and practices in the area of family living. Before any data on

One of the most
effective ways to assess
student progress toward
health literacy is to
observe whether their
behavior supports or
improves their health.

---

[2] *Education Code* Section 60800 requires school districts to administer a health-related physical fitness test to students in grades five, seven, and nine each year during March, April, or May.

student behavior are collected, schools should consider working with parents and local community organizations or agencies to provide education and information about the assessment, the rationale for the assessment design, and the intended use of the assessment data. This communication with parents and the community can help prevent misunderstandings and garner support for quality assessments.

In addition to using assessment results with individual students, teachers should use student assessment data to evaluate the overall health curriculum. The data can provide insights as to whether the curriculum is meeting the needs of all students, is building on prior knowledge appropriately, and is consistent with the developmental levels of the students.

Staff Assessment

Because health education involves staff not only as teachers but as adult models of good health, the attitudes and habits of staff members regarding health play an important role in promoting student health literacy. Voluntary assessments of staff health behaviors and attitudes about health, as well as approaches used to promote health literacy, will provide useful information about the staff's commitment to influencing students' health and incorporating health literacy into their own lives. The results will serve as a needs assessment for designing professional development activities.

Whatever the grade level, staff assessment and follow-up staff development workshops should be based on current information about health literacy and effective teaching methods. Pedagogical skills that support critical thinking and a student-centered curriculum are required to address the unifying ideas and expectations of this framework. Assessment should focus on the extent to which teaching strategies support students in developing the knowledge, skills, attitudes, and behaviors necessary to achieve health literacy. For example, assessments might ask teachers to reflect on how their teaching strategies help students (1) develop decision-making and thinking skills; (2) solve problems individually and as part of a group inquiry; and (3) gather, analyze, and present information. Teachers might also reflect on how they support the development of student health literacy by (1) connecting concepts in health education with learning in other curriculum areas; (2) cooperating with other school staff members to make student health literacy a priority at the school; and (3) considering the culture, ethnic values, and customs of the community in curriculum design and delivery.

How instructional strategies used by teachers and the health literacy of teachers are assessed will depend on the resources and staff available. Assessment can be done through anonymous questionnaires, self-studies, or observations. One or more designated staff members, preferably members of the school or school district health committee, should take the lead and have the knowledge and skills needed to carry out this responsibility. The information collected will help staff reflect on their practices and determine changes they can make to promote student health literacy.

System Assessment

Assessment of the coordinated school health system can provide invaluable information for planning program improvements to promote student health literacy. The assessment should involve both monitoring the implementation of a coordinated school health system and evaluating the influence of this system on student health literacy. It should involve collecting data on such factors as the following:

- Number of students participating in different aspects of the coordinated school health system, such as the number of students participating in planned, sequential health education and physical education
- Extent to which all the components of a coordinated school health system are being implemented[3]
- Levels of parent and community involvement
- Degree to which appropriate program planning has taken place
- Extent to which the school vision for the coordinated school health system has been articulated and the manner in which policies have been developed, reviewed, and implemented to support this vision
- Extent of linkages among the components of a coordinated school health system
- Extent to which health education has been infused into the other curriculum areas

The assessment should also examine the allocation of staff and resources to support the coordinated school health system. If available, community health data, such as the prevalence of iron-deficiency anemia among children, the number of accidents involving bicycles in the past year, the prevalence of sexually transmitted diseases among teenagers, or the incidence of teen pregnancy may be used together with school data. The assessment should be done in the initial planning stages and in each year thereafter so that schools can monitor their efforts to promote student health literacy and adjust those efforts as necessary to improve their effectiveness.

Using data from student, staff, and system assessments, the school should attempt to demonstrate, over a period of several years, the extent to which students have achieved health literacy and incorporated the values of that literacy into their daily living. Measuring the full continuum of outcomes, including positive changes in knowledge, attitudes, skills, and behaviors, will demand a variety of assessment methods and patience. Those planning assessments and using the assessment results must be mindful that change in behavior requires time. However, given the potential of assessment to influence long-term health behaviors of students, quality assessments must be developed and used to support progress toward health literacy for all students.

---

[3] See Chapter 1 for an explanation of the coordinated school health system.

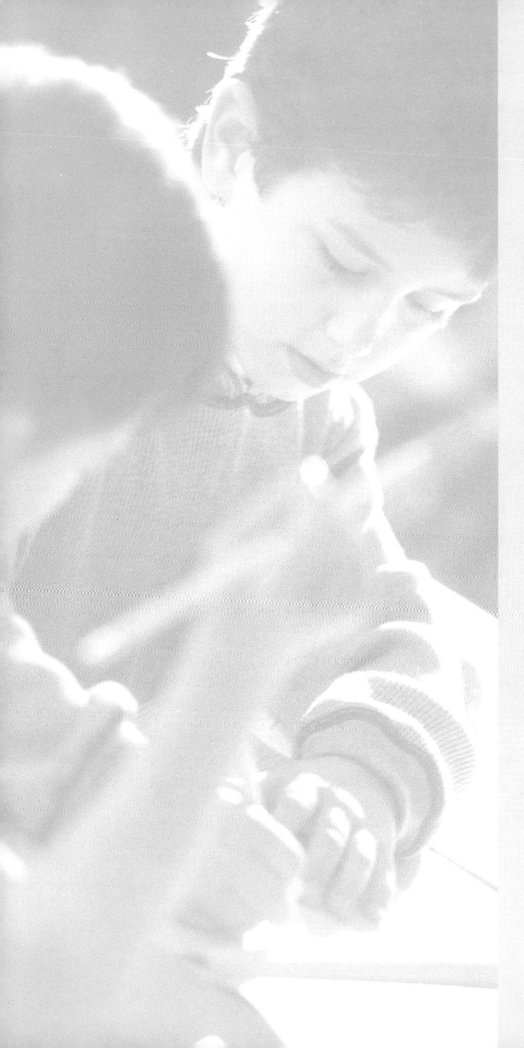

CHAPTER 6

Criteria for
Evaluating
Instructional
Materials for
Kindergarten
Through
Grade Eight

Chapter 6
Criteria for
Evaluating
Instructional
Materials for
Kindergarten
Through
Grade Eight

The criteria for evaluating the alignment of instructional materials with the content of the *Health Framework for California Public Schools, Kindergarten Through Grade Twelve* and evaluating the quality of those materials in the areas of grade-level emphases, curriculum content, program organization, assessment, universal access, and instructional planning and support are discussed in this section. These criteria will guide the development and govern the adoption in 2004 of instructional materials for kindergarten through grade eight. The criteria do not recommend nor require one particular pedagogical approach, nor does the numerical order of the criteria within each category imply relative importance. The criteria may also be used by publishers and local educational agencies as a guide for the development and selection of instructional materials for grades nine through twelve.

The criteria are organized into five categories:

1. **Health Content/Alignment with Curriculum:** The content as specified in the *Health Framework*
2. **Program Organization:** The sequence and organization of the health instructional materials
3. **Assessment:** The strategies presented in the instructional materials for measuring what students know and are able to do
4. **Universal Access:** The information and ideas that address the needs of special student populations, including students identified for special education, English learners, and advanced students
5. **Instructional Planning and Support:** The instructional planning and support information and materials, typically including a separate edition specially designed for use by the teacher, that assist teachers in the implementation of the health education program

Health materials must support teaching aligned with the *Health Framework.* Materials that fail to meet the health content criteria will not be considered satisfactory for adoption. Only programs that are determined to have met Criterion 1 will be further evaluated under Criteria 2 through 5.

In order to create focused health instructional materials, publishers are asked to concentrate on the content described in the *Health Framework,* especially in Chapter 3, "Health Education," and the Grade-Level Emphases Chart, as adopted by the State Board of Education in March 2002. The instructional materials must not contain extraneous content that is fundamentally contrary to the *Health Framework* and detracts from the ability of teachers to teach readily and students to learn thoroughly the content specified by the *Health Framework.*

CRITERION 1: HEALTH CONTENT/ALIGNMENT WITH CURRICULUM

Instructional materials support the teaching and learning of the skills and knowledge called for at the specific grade levels as outlined in the *Health*

223

Chapter 6
Criteria for
Evaluating
Instructional
Materials for
Kindergarten
Through
Grade Eight

Framework, including the emphases designated in the Grade-Level Emphases Chart. Materials are fully aligned with the framework content. Materials must be scientifically and medically accurate, must be based on current and confirmed research, and must enable students to develop goals of lifelong positive health behaviors and attitudes. Materials must meet all criteria. Materials with a glaring weakness or significant omission are not worthy of adoption. Programs with inaccuracies or errors that hinder the teaching of health content will not be considered for adoption. To be considered suitable for adoption, health instructional materials must provide:

1. Evidence and appropriate references, with page numbers, that demonstrate alignment with the Grade-Level Emphases Chart and content found in Chapter 3

2. Support of all content, as specified at each grade level, by topics, concepts, lessons, activities, examples, and/or illustrations, as appropriate

3. Integration and coordination with the eight components of coordinated school health[1] and support of the four unifying ideas of coordinated school health[2]

4. Accurate content to support health instruction as outlined in the *Health Framework* and in pertinent *Education Code* sections

5. Interesting and engaging health content that provides students with methods of evaluating the accuracy of health information claims through the use of scientific criteria and, when appropriate to the grade level, explains how to apply information to assess health-related behaviors

6. Medical and health vocabulary used appropriately and defined accurately

7. Scientifically and medically accurate content that reflects current practices in use or recommended by health professionals

8. Direct instruction and activities that focus on students improving and demonstrating proficiency in the topics noted in the Grade-Level Emphases Chart

9. Instruction that is appropriate to the grade level and develops health literacy (Health literacy is the capacity of an individual to obtain, interpret, and understand basic health information and services and the competence to use such information and services in ways that assist in maintaining and enhancing health.)

10. When appropriate, opportunities for students to increase their knowledge and understanding of health while reinforcing the skills and knowledge

---

[1] Health Education; Physical Education; Health Services; Nutrition Services; Psychological and Counseling Services; Health Promotion for Staff; Safe and Healthy School Environment; and Parent and Community Involvement (see Chapter 4, "Beyond Health Education").

[2] Acceptance of personal responsibility for lifelong health; Respect for and promotion of the health of others; An understanding of the process of growth and development; and Informed use of health-related information, products, and services (see Chapter 3, "Health Education"). Also important is reinforcing instruction on health behavior and health literacy through a collaborative effort by parents, the school, and the community.

224

Chapter 6
Criteria for
Evaluating
Instructional
Materials for
Kindergarten
Through
Grade Eight

called for in the physical education, reading/language arts, mathematics, science, history–social science, and visual and performing arts curriculum frameworks

11. When appropriate, opportunities for students to evaluate the accuracy of health-related information and to seek reputable resources and information

12. When called for by the Grade-Level Emphases Chart, introduction or review of topics that are emphasized at another grade level

13. Compliance with all relevant *Education Code* sections, including sections 233.5, 51201.5, 51240, 51513, 51550, and 51553–55

Materials being considered for adoption must meet Criterion 1 before being evaluated according to Criteria 2 through 5.

CRITERION 2: PROGRAM ORGANIZATION

The sequential organization of the health instructional materials provides structure for what students should learn at each grade level and allows teachers to convey the health content efficiently and effectively. The materials are well organized and presented in a manner that provides all students opportunities to acquire the essential knowledge and skills described in the *Health Framework.* Materials must designate which grade levels are being addressed. To be considered suitable for adoption, health instructional materials must provide:

1. Alignment with the *Health Framework,* introducing new knowledge and skills at a reasonable pace and depth of coverage and explicitly preparing students for later grade levels

2. Organization that provides a logical and coherent structure to facilitate efficient and effective teaching and learning within the lesson, unit, and grade level as described in the *Health Framework* and the Grade-Level Emphases Chart

3. Clearly stated student outcomes and goals that are measurable and are based on the framework

4. An overview of the content in each chapter or unit that designates how the lesson supports the *Health Framework*

5. A well-organized structure that provides students with the opportunity to learn the grade-level topics and build on knowledge and skills acquired at earlier grade levels

6. A variety of activities and texts that organize the grade-level content in a logical way so that students develop prerequisite skills and knowledge before they are introduced to the more complex concepts and understandings of the topic

7. Tables of contents, indexes, glossaries, content summaries, references, and assessment guides that are designed to help teachers, parents or guardians, and students use the materials

225

Chapter 6
Criteria for
Evaluating
Instructional
Materials for
Kindergarten
Through
Grade Eight

CRITERION 3: ASSESSMENT

Assessment should measure what students know and are able to do. Instructional materials should contain multiple measures to assess student progress. Assessment measures should reveal students' knowledge and understanding of the health content. Assessment tools that publishers include as part of their instructional material should provide evidence of students' progress toward meeting the skills and knowledge identified in the Grade-Level Emphases Chart. Assessment tools should provide information that teachers can use in planning and modifying instruction to help all students. To be considered suitable for adoption, health instructional materials must provide:

1. Strategies or instruments that teachers can use to determine students' prior knowledge
2. Multiple measures of individual student progress at regular intervals to evaluate attainment of grade-level knowledge, understanding, and ability to independently apply health concepts, principles, theories, and skills and to evaluate students' abilities to evaluate the accuracy of health-related information and to seek reputable resources and information
3. Guiding questions for monitoring student comprehension
4. Assessments that students can use to evaluate and improve the quality of their own work
5. Formative, summative, and cumulative assessments to evaluate students' work

CRITERION 4: UNIVERSAL ACCESS

Instructional materials should provide access to the curriculum for all students, including those with special needs: English learners, advanced learners, students with learning difficulties, special education students, and other students with special needs. Materials must conform to the policies of the State Board of Education as well as to other applicable state and federal guidelines pertaining to diverse populations and students with special needs. To be considered suitable for adoption, health instructional materials must provide:

1. Suggestions based on current and confirmed research for adapting the curriculum and the instruction to meet students' assessed special needs
2. Strategies to help students who are below grade level in reading, writing, speaking, and listening in English to understand the health content
3. Suggestions for advanced learners that are tied to the *Health Framework* and that allow students to study content in greater depth

CRITERION 5: INSTRUCTIONAL PLANNING AND SUPPORT

Support materials for teachers should be built into the instructional materials and should specify suggestions for and illustrate examples of how teachers can implement the *Health Framework* in a way that ensures an opportunity for all

Chapter 6
Criteria for
Evaluating
Instructional
Materials for
Kindergarten
Through
Grade Eight

students to learn the essential skills and knowledge called for in the *Health Framework,* including health literacy. These criteria do not recommend or require a particular pedagogical approach. Publishers should make recommendations to teachers regarding instructional approaches that fit the instructional goals. Materials should provide teachers with a variety of instructional approaches. To be considered suitable for adoption, planning and support resources must provide:

1. Clearly written and accurate explanations of health content, with suggestions for connecting health concepts with other areas of the curriculum

2. Strategies for addressing and correcting common misconceptions about health topics

3. A variety of pedagogical strategies

4. Lesson plans, suggestions for organizing resources in the classroom, and ideas for pacing lessons

5. Support for or access to confirmed, research-based programs

6. A list of materials, educational resources, and tools that align with the recommendations in the *Health Framework*

7. Suggestions and information for teachers to locate, interpret, convey, and apply medically and scientifically accurate content and current, confirmed research

8. Suggestions for how to use student assessment data within the program for instructional planning purposes

9. Technical support and suggestions for appropriate use of audiovisual, multimedia, and information technology resources associated with a unit

10. Suggestions for linking the classroom with reputable community resources in a manner consistent with state laws and school policies

11. Suggestions for activities and strategies for informing parents or guardians about the health program and creating connections among students, parents, guardians, and the community

12. References and resources to guide teachers' further study of health topics and suggestions

13. Demonstration of electronic resources (videos, DVDs, CDs) depicting appropriate teaching techniques and offering suggestions for teachers

14. Homework assignments that support classroom learning, give clear directions, and provide practice and reinforcement for the skills taught in the classroom

15. Suggestions for encouraging students to study content in greater depth

16. In the teacher's edition, ample and useful annotations and suggestions for presenting the content of the student edition and ancillary materials

Appendix A
Selected Legislative Code Sections

This section contains information primarily related to the *Education Code* and includes summaries of selected legislative code sections. The information was current at the time of publication; however, those using this section should keep in mind that the code sections might be amended by subsequent legislation. Educators and others interested in supporting coordinated school health are encouraged to keep up to date on legislative changes that affect students' health and health education.

Relevance of Legislation to Health Education

It is essential that California educators clearly understand the laws regarding their responsibility to protect and promote the health and safety of schoolchildren. Many laws are in effect that apply to multiple aspects of the delivery of health-related education, programs, and services. Selected legislative code sections cover the following topics:

- Specific content and delivery of instruction in the health curriculum
- Requirements for parent notification and community involvement in school health programs
- Specific training requirements for those who provide instruction in health or health services at the school site
- Mandates on how to deal with potential student health problems, safety risks, confidentiality, and crisis intervention
- Requirements for protecting students' health and safety

This document provides an overview of school health laws in effect at the time of publication. For up-to-date information about school health laws in California, consult the following Web sites:

- California Healthy Kids
  <http://www.californiahealthykids.org>
  This Web site provides an online database of edited school health laws. From this site users can obtain the text of a single law or a custom list of selected laws.
- California Law
  <http://www.leginfo.ca.gov/calaw.html>
  This Web site provides the full legal text of each law. This site also offers the option of subscribing to updates on bills as they pass through the legislative process. Subscribers receive notification when legislative action is taken on a bill.

Organization of Health-Related Code Sections

Many sections of the *Education Code* (and sections of other legislation) relate to health instruction and the components of a coordinated school health system. Such sections are dispersed throughout the *Education Code.* The relevant legislative sections have been organized in tables as follows to facilitate user reference:

- Table A.1, "Health Education Mandates." Indicates the mandates for health education. Summaries of code sections cited in this table may be found after Table A.3.
- Table A.2, "Health Education Recommendations." Indicates laws that encourage or recommend topics and priorities for health education instruction.
- Table A.3, "Coordinated School Health Legislation." Briefly describes many of the laws related to the other components of a coordinated school health system.

Table A.1 Health Education Mandates

	Instruction	*Teacher Preparation Requirements*	*Parent Notification/ Community Involvement*	*Materials*
Comprehensive Health Education	*EC* 51202 *EC* 51210(f) *EC* 51880– 81.5(b) *EC* 51890 *EC* 51911 *EC* 51913–14		*PC* 11166(a) *EC* 51513	*EC* 51891 *EC* 60040–42 *EC* 60044
Alcohol, Tobacco, and Other Drugs	*EC* 51202–03 *EC* 51260–66.5 *EC* 51268–69	*EC* 51260–66.5 *EC* 51268–69	*HSC* 11802	
HIV/AIDS, STDs	*EC* 51201.5 (a),(b) *EC* 51554(a)	*EC* 51229.8	*EC* 51201.5 (a),(b) *EC* 51240 *EC* 51555	
Family Life/ Sex Education	*EC* 51553(a) *EC* 51554(a)		*EC* 51240 *EC* 51550 *EC* 51555	
Pregnancy/ Parenting Education	*EC* 51220.5(c)			
Violence Prevention, Safety	*EC* 233.5(a) *EC* 35294	*GC* 3100		

Key: Education Code (EC); Government Code (GC); Health and Safety Code (HSC); Penal Code (PC).

Table A.2   Health Education Recommendations

	Instruction	Teacher Preparation Requirements	Parent Notification/ Community Involvement	Materials
Comprehensive Health Education				EC 60042
Alcohol, Tobacco, and Other Drugs	EC 51262	EC 44645		
HIV/AIDS, STDs	EC 51820		EC 51820	
Family Life/ Sex Education	EC 51553			
Pregnancy/ Parenting Education	EC 8910–11			
Violence Prevention, Safety	EC 51860	EC 51265		
Environmental Protection	EC 8700–07 EC 8720–23			

Note: Text from the *Education Code* regarding "recommendations" for health instruction and coordinated school health is not included in this appendix because of space limitations. A summary of the text can be viewed on the Web at <*http://www.californiahealthykids.org*>. The full text can be viewed at <*http:// www.leginfo.ca.gov/calaw.html*>.

Coordinated School Health Legislation

Beyond the Health Education component of a coordinated school health system are seven additional components, described in Chapter 4, "Beyond Health Education." Several of those components—Physical Education, Health Services, Nutrition Services, and Psychological and Counseling Services—are supported by the *Education Code* sections cited in Table A.3.

Table A.3 Coordinated School Health Legislation

CSH Component	Laws and Regulations	Topic
Physical Education	EC 51206	Requires the State Superintendent of Public Instruction to employ a physical education specialist to develop curriculum and staff development.
	EC 51220–22	Require student participation in physical education.
	EC 51225.3	Requires two physical education courses during grades 9–12 for graduation. (Requires a minimum of 400 minutes for every 10 school days.)
	EC 51210, 51223	Require physical education for elementary students for a minimum of 200 minutes for every 10 school days.
	EC 60800	Requires annual physical fitness testing for grades 5, 7, and 9.
	EC 52715	Requires school districts to employ teachers with physical education certification qualifications.
Health Services	EC 49427	Directs local educational agency (LEA) administrators to maintain fundamental school health services at a specified minimum level.
	CCR, Title 17, 6802; HSC 124085	Require a Child Health Disability Prevention physical examination in grade 1.
	EC 48211–13, 48980, 49403, 49450–51; CCR, Title 17, 2506; CCR, Title 5, 202	Include requirements for communicable disease control measures.
	HSC 120335	Includes required immunizations for school entry.
	EC 49451	Gives parents the right to refuse consent to health screenings.
	EC 49452.5	Requires scoliosis screening.
	EC 49450	Requires confidentiality of health screening records.
	EC 49456	Requires schools to report to parents on health screening results.
	USC, Title 20, 1400	Requires education for all disabled children.

Note: Text from the laws and regulations cited here is not included in this appendix because of space limitations. Summaries of the text from California laws can be viewed on the Web at <http://www.californiahealthykids.org>. The full text can be viewed at <http://www.leginfo.ca.gov/calaw.html>.

Key: California Code of Regulations (CCR); Education Code (EC); Health and Safety Code (HSC); United States Code (USC).

Table A.3 Coordinated School Health Legislation (Continued)

CSH Component	Laws and Regulations	Topic
Health Services (*Continued*)	*CCR, Title 5*, 3001, 3021.1	Require referral for chronic illness.
	EC 49452; *CCR, Titles 5* and *17*	Include requirements for vision and hearing screenings and referrals.
Nutrition Services	*EC* 499530–36	Set proper nutrition as a high priority. LEAs may apply to CDE for available state and local funds for breakfast and lunch programs.
	EC 49500–05	Set forth legislative intent that no child is to go hungry.
	EC 49590	Allows LEAs to authorize food sale on school premises.
	EC 49490–96	Establish nutrition services standards.
	EC 49510–20	Set forth intent that students who receive public assistance are ensured of a supplemental food program while they attend school.
	EC 49530	Establishes nutritional requirements for foods sold at elementary and secondary schools (SB 19, Pupil Nutrition, Health, and Achievement Act of 2001).
	EC 49547–48	Discuss summer meal service.
Psychological and Counseling Services	*EC* 49424	Defines school psychologist services by a credentialed school psychologist.
	EC 49600	Defines "educational counseling" services and programs to be provided by credentialed school counselors.
	EC 49602	Defines students' rights to confidentiality and lists provisions for reporting confidential information.

Summaries of Selected *Education Code* Sections

Education Code Section 233.5(a), principals of morality

Teachers shall endeavor to impress upon the minds of students the principles of morality, truth, justice, citizenship, and so forth.

Education Code Section 35294, programs for school safety and violence prevention

California public schools should develop for kindergarten through grade twelve a comprehensive school safety plan that addresses safety concerns that are identified through a systematic planning process.

Education Code sections 51201.5(a) and 51201.5(b), instruction on the prevention of AIDS

School districts shall ensure that all students in grades seven through twelve receive instruction on AIDS prevention. Each student shall receive the instruction at least once in junior high or middle school and once in high school. Parent notification of such instruction is required.

Education Code Section 51202, instruction on personal and public health and safety

The adopted course of study shall provide, in the appropriate elementary and secondary grades, instruction on first aid, fire prevention, conservation of resources, and health, including the effects of alcohol, drugs, and so forth.

Education Code Section 51203, instruction on alcohol, narcotics, restricted dangerous drugs, and so forth

Instruction on the nature of alcohol, narcotics, restricted dangerous drugs, and so forth shall be provided in elementary and secondary schools. Governing boards shall adopt regulations specifying the grade levels and the courses in which such instruction is provided.

Education Code Section 51210(f), instruction in areas of study

The adopted course of study in grades one through six shall include health instruction, including instruction on the principles and practices of individual, family, and community health.

Education Code Section 51220.5(c), parenting skills

The adopted course of study for grade seven or eight shall include the equivalent content of a one-semester course in parenting education and skills so that students will acquire basic knowledge of parenting.

Education Code Section 51229.8, in-service training on AIDS-prevention instruction

County offices of education and school districts, through regional training, shall plan and conduct in-service training for all teachers and school employees who provide AIDS-prevention instruction.

Education Code Section 51240, written request by parent to excuse student from family life/sex education

A parent or guardian may request that a student be excused from family life/sex education when such instruction conflicts with religious beliefs and training.

Education Code Section 51260, trained instructors for drug education

Instructors in drug education, which includes the effects of the use of tobacco, alcohol, narcotics, dangerous drugs, and so forth, must be appropriately trained.

Education Code Section 51261, approval and reevaluation of teacher certification programs for drug education

The State Board of Education shall approve only those teacher certification programs for drug education that qualify under this section and shall continually reevaluate those programs.

Education Code Section 51262, instruction on the use of anabolic steroids

A lesson on the effects of the use of anabolic steroids should be included in science, health, drug abuse, or physical education programs in grades seven through twelve.

Education Code Section 51263, information on programs for the prevention of drug and alcohol abuse

The California Department of Education shall make available information on model drug- and alcohol-abuse prevention education programs developed and funded by state and federal agencies.

Education Code sections 51264(a) and 51264(d), in-service training on the prevention of gang violence and drug and alcohol abuse

The California Department of Education shall prepare and distribute to school districts and county offices of education guidelines for incorporating into staff development plans in-service training for teachers, counselors, athletic directors, and so forth on the prevention of gang violence and drug and alcohol abuse. Each school is encouraged to develop a single plan to strengthen its efforts to prevent gang violence and drug and alcohol abuse and to include these topics in its school improvement or school safety plan.

Education Code Section 51265, priority of in-service training on the prevention of gang violence and drug and alcohol abuse

School districts and county offices of education should give a high priority to in-service training programs for comprehensive gang-violence and drug- and alcohol-abuse prevention education.

Education Code Section 51266(a), curriculum for the prevention of gang violence and substance abuse

The Office of Criminal Justice Planning and the California Department of Education shall collaborate to develop a model curriculum for the suppression of gang violence and the prevention of substance abuse for grades two, four, and six.

Education Code Section 51266.5, model curriculum for the prevention of gang violence and substance abuse

State agencies shall review the model curriculum for gang-violence suppression and substance-abuse prevention for grades two, four, and six and shall identify the methods by which the curriculum can be most fully implemented in rural school settings.

Education Code Section 51268, duplication of efforts in the prevention of drug, alcohol, and tobacco abuse

The California Department of Education shall offer to school districts and county offices of education guidance on avoiding duplication of efforts in the administration of education programs for the prevention of drug, alcohol, and tobacco abuse.

Education Code sections 51269(a) and 51269(b), improved delivery of programs for the prevention of drug, alcohol, and tobacco abuse

The California Department of Education shall, to the extent possible, collaborate with other state agencies that administer education programs for the prevention of drug, alcohol, and tobacco abuse to streamline and simplify funding application processes. The Department shall develop an ongoing, statewide monitoring, assessment, and data collection system to improve program planning and delivery.

Education Code Section 51513, questions asked of students

Parents and guardians must be notified in writing of any test, questionnaire, survey, or examination to be administered that contains questions regarding beliefs and practices in sex, family life, morality, and religion.

Education Code Section 51550, parent notification of family life and sex education courses

Governing boards of public schools may not require students to attend any class in which reproductive organs and their functions and processes are described, illustrated, or discussed. If such classes are offered, parents and guardians of all students must be notified in writing.

Education Code Section 51553(a), sex education course criteria

All classes in grades one through twelve that teach sex education and discuss sexual intercourse shall emphasize abstinence from sexual intercourse as the only protection that is 100 percent effective against unintended pregnancy, STDs, and AIDS.

Education Code Section 51554(a), parent notification of instruction on family life, AIDS, STDs, and so forth

Parents and guardians shall be notified in writing at the beginning of the school year (or at the time of enrollment when a student enrolls after the beginning of the school year) of any instruction on family life, AIDS, STDs, and so forth that will be delivered by an outside organization or guest speaker brought in specifically to provide that instruction.

Education Code Section 51555, instruction on family life, AIDS, STDs, and so forth in kindergarten through grade six

School districts, county boards of education, or county superintendents of schools shall provide parents and guardians of all students written notice that instruction on family life, AIDS, STDs, and so forth will be given. Information stating parents' and guardians' right to request copies of sections 51201.5 and 51553 (relating to AIDS-prevention instruction) shall be included in the written notice.

Education Code Section 51880, Comprehensive Health Education Act of 1977

An adequate health education program in the public schools is essential to continued progress and improvement in the quality of public health in California. Maximum use shall be made of existing state and federal funds in the implementation of comprehensive health education.

Education Code Section 51881.5(b), hazardous substances

Hazardous substances education programs in public schools are beneficial, fostering in students an understanding of their role in protecting the environment and in safeguarding themselves from the dangers posed by hazardous substances.

Education Code Section 51890, comprehensive health education programs

Comprehensive health education programs are defined as all educational programs offered in kindergarten through grade twelve that are designed to ensure that students will receive instruction that helps them in their decision making regarding personal, family, and community health.

Education Code Section 51891, community participation in comprehensive health education

The planning, implementation, and evaluation of comprehensive health education must include active community participation.

Education Code Section 51911, evaluation of comprehensive health education programs

Approval of district plans shall be made in accordance with rules and regulations adopted by the State Board of Education.

Education Code Section 51913, evaluation standards and criteria

The State Board of Education shall establish standards and criteria to be used in the evaluation of plans for comprehensive health education programs submitted by school districts to the State Board for approval.

Education Code Section 51914, cooperation of parents, community, and teachers in the development of health education programs

Comprehensive health education programs must be developed with the active cooperation of parents, the community, and teachers in all stages of planning, approval, and implementation.

Education Code Section 60040, adoption of instructional materials that portray diversity

All instructional materials adopted by governing boards shall accurately portray the cultural and racial diversity of our society.

Education Code Section 60041, adoption of instructional materials that portray humanity's place in ecological systems

Instructional materials adopted by governing boards shall accurately portray, whenever appropriate, humanity's place in ecological systems and the necessity of protecting the environment.

Education Code Section 60042, adoption of instructional materials that encourage responsible behaviors

Adopted instructional materials must encourage thrift, fire prevention, and the humane treatment of animals and people.

Education Code Section 60044, prohibited instructional materials

No instructional materials shall be adopted that reflect adversely on people because of their race, color, creed, national origin, ancestry, sex, disability, or occupation.

Summaries of Other Selected Legislative Code Sections

Government Code Section 3100, public employees as disaster service workers

All public employees are declared to be disaster service workers for the protection of citizens' health, safety, lives, and property in the event of disasters bought about by natural, man-made, or war-caused emergencies.

Health and Safety Code Section 11802(a), funds for alcohol-abuse prevention programs

Funds shall be allocated to programs for alcohol-abuse prevention in schools and the community.

Penal Code Section 11166(a), reporting of child abuse

"Mandated reporters" (defined in Section 11165.7 to include teachers, instructional aides, classified school employees, and so forth) who know of or reasonably suspect child abuse shall report the known or suspected instance to a child protection agency immediately or as soon as is practicably possible.

Appendix B

Project TEACH Recommendations on Preservice Teacher Training in Health Education

Project TEACH, funded by the California Department of Education and College Health 2000, was designed to improve preservice teacher training in health education. All colleges and universities providing teacher training in California were invited to participate. The project examined current practices and collaboratively developed recommendations. These recommendations, issued in 1993, are being used by participating institutions to help new teachers promote health literacy among their students more effectively. The Project TEACH recommendations, exemplary only, are presented as follows: [1]

1. Universities/colleges should offer two separate courses—one for single-subject credential candidates (secondary) and one for multiple-subject credential candidates (elementary).

2. The courses should each be three units (semester or quarter) in length, and there should be a minimum of 40 to 50 contact hours between the students and the instructor.

3. Challenges to the course (credit by examination) should not be allowed. Students should receive credit for the course only by completing the course requirements.

4. CPR certification must cover infant-child and adult CPR as well as choking emergencies (American Red Cross Community CPR or American Heart Association B-level).

5. Instructors are expected to utilize the *Health Framework* and familiarize the students with mandated areas of instruction and *Education Code* sections related to health education.

6. The courses should deal primarily with the health status and health instruction of children and adolescents. A personal health and wellness text (of the type used in introductory college personal health courses) is *not* appropriate for use in these teacher education courses.

7. The course for the multiple-subject (elementary) teachers should:

   a. Make prospective teachers aware of health issues related to children.
   b. Make prospective teachers aware of the structure of a comprehensive school health system.

---

[1] For more information contact Deborah Wood, Director, Healthy Kids Resource Center, Alameda County Office of Education.

Appendix B
Project TEACH
Recommendations
on Preservice
Teacher Training in
Health Education

    c. Help prospective teachers become familiar with the materials and methods used in comprehensive school health education.

    d. Utilize a variety of instructional strategies to model possible health education strategies.

    e. Include use of an appropriate text and/or instructional materials that will enable students to become familiar with lesson plans, resources for health education, instructional techniques, and the like.

    f. Acquaint prospective teachers with the year 2000 objectives that affect K–6 students and the health emphasis of *It's Elementary.*

8. The course for single-subject (secondary) teachers should:

    a. Acquaint prospective teachers with the year 2000 objectives for students in grades seven through twelve and the health emphasis of *Second to None.*

    b. Make prospective teachers aware of the structure of a comprehensive school health system.

    c. Teach prospective teachers how to integrate health instruction into their single-subject curriculum.

    d. Acquaint prospective teachers with the health problems and concerns of adolescents. Included are such topics as teenage pregnancy, acne, sexually transmitted diseases, steroids, substance abuse, abusive relationships, mental health, injury prevention, and nutrition.

    e. Emphasize the relationship between health and student performance.

9. Rename poorly named courses to reflect *what should be taught* in the course. Suggested course names may include:

Health Education for Elementary Teachers

Health Education for Secondary Teachers

Some course titles that would *not* be appropriate are Personal Health, Contemporary Health Issues, Health, Substance Abuse and Nutrition Education, Health and Hygiene, Nutrition, Fitness, Biology, and Health Studies.

10. Students who take a personal health course at a junior college or at another school should not be allowed to have that course fill the obligation for the health education for teachers requirement. Universities should instruct their credential analyst to require students to take the specific course in health education for teachers.

11. When universities offer only the combined course (for both multiple- and single-subject teachers), care must be taken that multiple-subject teachers are trained in content and teaching methods. Single-subject teachers must be trained in how to infuse/integrate their curriculum with health topics. This becomes a difficult task with the limited class time available. For this reason, recommendation 1 should be given top priority.

Appendix C

Guidelines for Evaluating Web Sites

Growing numbers of Americans are turning to the Internet to obtain health-related information. Those numbers increasingly include educators who specialize in school health.

The availability of almost unlimited information is one of the great advantages of the World Wide Web, but the Web also poses a potential problem, especially regarding health-related information. "With a click of the mouse," observed the International Food Information Council in 1999, "a word-of-mouth phenomenon can be multiplied exponentially via the World Wide Web or electronic mail and result in questionable nutrition, food, safety, and health stories being sent directly to your computer."[1] Researchers Kotecki and Chamness emphasize that "To ensure proper information use, consumers must be able to separate credible WWW sites from noncredible sites."[2]

One way to evaluate Web sites is through online reviews and discussions with other school health professionals. Another is to bookmark Web sites that have proven reliable in the past and to refer primarily to those sites and recommended links found on those sites. Several other guidelines can be helpful when reviewing Web sites:

- Be wary of Web sites that are designed primarily to promote or sell products and programs.
- Look beyond personal anecdotes and isolated examples; solid empirical research is preferable.
- Make sure to identify the source of the information. Established organizations and governmental agencies are likely to be more reliable than unknown or unrecognizable sources. Web sites ending in ".gov" or ".edu," for example, are developed by official governmental and educational organizations.
- Note that the Healthy Kids Resource Center updates and evaluates the Web sites included in its "Links" list on a regular basis (<*http:// www.californiahealthykids.org*>).
- Maintain a questioning attitude; do not take information at face value.
- Be sure to refer to the *Getting Results* criteria for evaluating research-based practices when researching curriculum or programs (see Chapter 2, "Developing Health Literacy in the Classroom and in the School," in this framework).

The form that follows is an evaluation tool designed to help users of Web sites make well-informed decisions about a Web site's accuracy and utility.

---

[1] "The Mouse That Roared: Health Scares on the Internet," *Food Insight: Current Topics in Food Safety and Nutrition* (May/June 1999), 1–5.

[2] J. E. Kotecki and B. E. Chamness, "A Valid Tool for Evaluating Health-Related WWW Sites," *Journal of Health Education,* Vol. 30, No. 1 (1999), 26-29.

Health-Related WWW Site Evaluation Tool

Title: _____

URL: http:// _____

Date: _____

Evaluator: _____

INFORMATION	Y	N
Criterion 1: Scope		
A. Many different aspects of the topic are presented.		
B. Each aspect is presented in depth.		
Criterion 2: Accuracy		
A. The information is consistent with other resources on the topic.		
B. The information presented is properly referenced.		
C. The information is based on scientific data published in peer-reviewed journals		
D. The site includes a disclaimer.		
Criterion 3: Authority		
A. The authors or organizations supplying the information are identified.		
B. The authors or organizations are recognized in the field.		
C. The credentials of the authors are identified.		
D. The authors are writing about their discipline.		
Criterion 4: Currency		
A. The information presented is up-to-date.		
B. The information builds on previous knowledge.		
Criterion 5: Purpose		
A. The purpose of the site is identified.		
B. The information is appropriate for the intended purpose.		
C. The intended audience is specified.		
D. The source of funding for the site is identified.		

DESIGN	Y	N
Criterion 6: Organization, Structure, and Design		
A. The information presented in the site is well-organized.		
B. The terminology used is meaningful to the subject area.		
C. The site contains a table of contents or provides an organizational structure that makes the content easy to access.		
D. The site contains specific links to data references.		
E. The site contains internal search engines.		
F. The document has a distinguishable header and footer.		
G. The major headings and subheadings are identifiable.		
H. The loading time for the site is reasonable.		
I. The site's creation date is clearly displayed.		
J. The date of the last revision is clearly displayed.		
K. The reading level and material presented is appropriate for the intended audience.		

Adapted from J. E. Kotecki, and B. E. Chamness, "A Valid Tool for Evaluating Health-Related WWW Sites," *Journal of Health Education*, Vol. 30, No. 1 (1999), 56–59.

Suggestions for rating: Tally the number of Y's for both major categories and rate the site by using the following scale:

Information
   13–16: Credible site: convincing evidence exists
    7–12: Ambivalent site: inconclusive evidence exists
     0–6: Red flag site: insufficient evidence exists

Design
    6–11: Accommodating site: easy to navigate
    0–5: Hindering site: difficult to navigate

Works Cited

Adelman, Howard. "School Counseling, Psychological, and Social Services," in *Health Is Academic: A Guide to Coordinated School Health Programs.* Edited by Eva Marx, Susan Frelick Wooley, and Daphne Northrop. New York: Teachers College Press, 1998.

"American Diabetes Association Position Statement: Care of Children with Diabetes in the School and Day Care Setting," *Diabetes Care,* Vol. 25 (2002), S122–26.

Araujo, D. "Expecting Questions About Exercise and Pregnancy?" *The Physician and Sportsmedicine,* Vol. 25, No. 4 (1997), 85–93.

Assessing Health Literacy: Assessment Framework. Prepared by the Council of Chief State School Officers. Soquel, Calif.: ToucanEd Publications, 1998.

Bandura, A. *Social Foundations of Thought and Action.* Englewood Cliffs, N.J.: Prentice Hall, 1986.

Baranowski, T.; C. L. Perry; and G. S. Parcel. "How Individual Environments and Health Behavior Interact: Social Cognitive Theory," in *Health Behavior and Health Education.* Edited by K. Glanz, F. M. Lewis, and B. K. Riner. San Francisco: Jossey-Bass, Inc., 1997.

Benard, Bonnie. "Resiliency Study," in *Getting Results, Part I: California Action Guide to Creating Safe and Drug-Free Schools and Communities.* Sacramento: California Department of Education, 1998. Citing Emmy E. Werner and Ruth S. Smith. *Overcoming the Odds: High-Risk Children from Birth to Adulthood.* New York: Cornell University Press, 1992.

Benard, Bonnie. "Resiliency Study," in *Getting Results, Part 1: California Action Guide to Creating Safe and Drug-Free Schools and Communities.* Sacramento: California Department of Education, 1998. Citing Emmy E. Werner and Ruth S. Smith. *Vulnerable but Invincible: A Longitudinal Study of Resilient Children and Youth.* New York: Adams, Bannister, and Cox, 1989.

Benson, Peter L. "Promoting Positive Human Development: The Power of Schools," in *Getting Results, Update 1: Positive Youth Development: Research, Commentary, and Action.* Sacramento: California Department of Education, 1999.

The Best Intentions: Unintended Pregnancy and the Well-Being of Children and Families. Edited by S. Brown and L. Eisenberg. Washington, D.C.: National Academic Press, 1995.

Botvin, G. J., and E. M. Botvin. "Adolescent Tobacco, Alcohol, and Drug Abuse: Prevention Strategies, Empirical Findings, and Assessment Issues," *Journal of Developmental and Behavioral Pediatrics,* Vol. 13 (1992), 291–301.

Bruvold, W. H. "A Meta-Analysis of Adolescent Smoking Prevention Programs," *American Journal of Public Health,* Vol. 83 (1993), 872–80.

The California Daily Food Guide. Developed by the California Department of Health Services in collaboration with the California Department of Aging and the California Department of Education. Sacramento: California Department of Education, 1990.

California Healthy Kids Survey. Sacramento: California Department of Education, 1999.

California Safe Schools Assessment: Promoting Safe Schools—1998-99 Results. Prepared by the California Department of Education, the Butte County Office of Education, and Duerr Evaluation Resources. Sacramento: California Department of Education, 2000.

Caught in the Middle: Educational Reform for Young Adolescents in California Public Schools. Sacramento: California Department of Education, 1987.

Choose Well, Be Well. Series of nutrition curriculum materials for students in preschool through grade twelve. Sacramento: California Department of Education, 1982–84.

Chronic Disease and Health Promotion: Reprints from the MMWR 1990–1991 Youth Risk Behavior Surveillance System. Atlanta: Centers for Disease Control and Prevention, n.d.

A Composite of Laws, California Special Education Programs, 25th Edition. Sacramento: California Department of Education, 2003.

Connell, D., and others. "Summary of Findings of the School Health Education Evaluation: Health Promotion Effectiveness, Implementation, and Costs," *Journal of School Health,* Vol. 55, No. 8 (1985), 316–21.

Donaldson, S. I., and others. "Resistance Skill Training and Onset of Alcohol Use: Evidence for Beneficial and Potentially Harmful Effects in Public and in Private Catholic Schools," *Health Psychology,* Vol. 14 (1995), 291–300.

Dwyer, K., and D. Osher. *Safeguarding Our Children: An Action Guide.* Washington, D.C.: U.S. Department of Education and U.S. Department of Justice, American Institutes for Research, 2000.

Dwyer, K.; D. Osher; and C. Warger. *Early Warning, Timely Response: A Guide to Safe Schools.* Washington, D.C.: U.S. Department of Education, 1998.

Eastin, Delaine. *A Report to the Legislature.* Sacramento: California Department of Education, 1996.

Enrolling Students Living in Homeless Situations. Sacramento: California Department of Education, 1999.

Family and Community Involvement: School Health Advisory Councils. Prepared by the California Center for Health Improvement, Sacramento, 2000.

Flay, B. R. "Psychosocial Approaches to Smoking Prevention: A Review of Findings," *Health Psychology,* Vol. 4, No. 5 (1985), 449–88.

Getting Results, Update 1: Positive Youth Development: Research, Commentary, and Action. Sacramento: California Department of Education, 1999.

Guide for Preventing and Responding to School Violence. Prepared by the Security Research Center. Alexandria, Va.: Association of Chiefs of Police Private Sector Liaison Committee, 2001.

Guidelines for School-Based Suicide Prevention Programs. Washington, D.C.: American Association of Suicidology, 1999.

Haggerty, R. J., and P. J. Mrazek. "Can We Prevent Mental Illness?" *Bulletin of the New York Academy of Medicine,* Vol. 71, No. 2 (1994), 300–06.

Hansen, W. B., and R. B. McNeal. "Drug Education Practice: Results of an Observational Study," *Health Education Research: Theory and Practice,* Vol. 14, No. 1 (1999), 85–97.

Hate-Motivated Behavior in Schools: Response Strategies for School Boards, Administrators, Law Enforcement, and Communities. Prepared by the Alameda County Office of Education and the California Department of Education. Sacramento: California Department of Education, 1997.

Health Is Academic: A Guide to Coordinated School Health Programs. Edited by Eva Marx, Susan Frelick Wooley, and Daphne Northrop. New York: Teachers College Press, 1998.

The Health of America's Children. Washington, D.C.: Children's Defense Fund, 1992.

Here They Come: Ready or Not! Report of the School Readiness Task Force. Sacramento: California Department of Education, 1988.

Herman, Joan L.; Lynn Lyons Morris, and Carol Taylor Fitz-Gibbon. *Evaluator's Handbook.* Newbury Park, Calif.: Sage Publications, 1987.

Homans, G. C. *Elementary Forms of Social Behavior* (Second edition). New York: Harcourt Brace Jovanovich, 1974.

Improving School Health: A Guide to School Health Councils. Developed by Christin P. Bellian. Atlanta: American Cancer Society, 1999.

Information Power: Building Partnerships for Learning. Chicago: American Library Association, 1998.

Involving the Family in School Health Advisory Councils. Prepared by the California Center for Health Improvement, Sacramento, 2000.

It's Elementary! Elementary Grades Task Force Report. Sacramento: California Department of Education, 1992.

James, B., and others. *Pieces of the Puzzle: Creating Success for Students in Homeless Situations.* Austin: University of Texas, 1997.

Keeping Schools Safe: Involving Parents and Other Caring Adults in Supervision Programs. Sacramento: Sacramento County Office of Education, 1999.

Kirby, D., and others. "Reducing the Risk : Impact of a New Curriculum on Sexual Risk-Taking," *Journal of School Health,* Vol. 23, No. 6 (1991), 253–63.

Kotecki, J. E., and B. E. Chamness. "A Valid Tool for Evaluating Health-Related WWW Sites," *Journal of Health Education,* Vol. 30, No. 1 (1999), 26–29.

Lantz, P. M., and others. "Investing in Youth Tobacco Control: A Review of Smoking Prevention and Control Strategies," *Tobacco Control,* Vol. 9 (2000), 47–63.

Laracy, M.; J. Levin-Epstein; and C. Shapiro. *Learning to Work Together: How Education and Welfare Agencies Can Coordinate Schooling/Training of AFDC Teen Parents.* Washington, D.C.: Center for Law and Social Policy, 1994.

Lindsay, J., and S. G. Enright. *Books, Babies and School-Age Parents: How to Teach Pregnant and Parenting Teens to Succeed.* Buena Park, Calif.: Morning Glory Press, 1997.

Managing Asthma in the School Environment. Washington, D.C.: U.S. Environmental Protection Agency, 2000.

McGuire, W. "Social Psychology," in *New Horizons in Psychology.* Edited by P. C. Dodwell. Middlesex, England: Penguin Books, 1972.

"The Mouse That Roared: Health Scares on the Internet," *Food Insight: Current Topics in Food Safety and Nutrition* (May/June 1999), 1–5.

National Association of School Nurses Position Statement: Caseload Assignments. National Association of School Nurses Web site *<http://208.5.177.157/ positions/caseload.htm>.* 1995.

National Mortality Statistics. Centers for Disease Control and Prevention Web site *<http://www.cdc.gov/ncipc>.* 2000.

National Strategy for Suicide Prevention: Goals and Objectives for Action. Washington, D.C.: U.S. Department of Health and Human Services, 2001.

1999 Annual Report on School Safety. Washington, D.C.: U.S. Department of Education and U.S. Department of Justice, 2000.

1996 Atlas of Births to California Teenagers. Sacramento: California Department of Health Services, 1998.

Not Schools Alone: Guidelines for Schools and Communities to Prevent the Use of Tobacco, Alcohol, and Other Drugs Among Children and Youth. Sacramento: California Department of Education, 1991.

Novello, A. C., and others. "Healthy Children Ready to Learn: An Essential Collaboration Between Health and Education," *Public Health Reports,* Vol. 107, No. 1 (1992), 3–14.

Nutrition Management of the Pregnant Adolescent: A Practical Reference Guide. Washington, D.C.: March of Dimes Birth Defects Foundation, 1990.

Nutritional Guide for Pregnant and Lactating Adolescents. Sacramento: California Department of Education, 1987.

On Alert! Gang Prevention: School In-Service Guidelines. Sacramento: California Department of Education, 1994.

O'Toole, Mary Ellen. *The School Shooter: A Threat Assessment Perspective.* Quantico, Va.: Federal Bureau of Investigation, 2000.

Perry, C. L., and S. H. Kelder. "Models for Effective Prevention," *Journal of Adolescent Health,* Vol. 13, No. 5 (1992), 355–63.

Physical Education Framework for California Public Schools, Kindergarten Through Grade Twelve. Sacramento: California Department of Education, 1994.

Policy: Adolescent Pregnancy and Parenting. Sacramento: California Department of Education, 1993.

Promoting Health Education in Schools: A Critical Issues Report. Arlington, Va.: American Association of School Administrators, 1985.

Reddy, M., and others. "Evaluating Risk for Targeted Violence in Schools: Comparing Risk Assessment, Threat Assessment, and Other Approaches," *Psychology in the Schools,* Vol. 38, No. 2 (2001), 157–72.

"Report of the 1990 Joint Committee on Health Education Terminology," *Journal of Health Education,* Vol. 22, No. 2 (1991), 104.

"Research into Action: Action Steps for Schools," in *Getting Results, Update 1: Positive Youth Development: Research, Commentary, and Action.* Sacramento: California Department of Education, 1999.

Resnick, Michael D. "Resiliency, Protective Factors, and Connections That Count in the Lives of Adolescents," in *Getting Results, Update 1: Positive Youth Development: Research, Commentary, and Action.* Sacramento: California Department of Education, 1999. Citing Milbrey W. McLaughlin and others. *Urban Sanctuaries: Neighborhood Organizations in the Lives and Futures of Inner-City Youth.* San Francisco: Jossey-Bass, Inc., 1994.

Resolutions and Policy Statements. Scarborough, Me.: National Association of School Nurses, 1990.

Safe Schools: A Planning Guide for Action. Prepared by the California Department of Education and the Office of the Attorney General. Sacramento: California Department of Education, 1995.

Sarvela, Paul D., and Robert J. McDermott. *Health Education Evaluation and Measurement: A Practitioner's Perspective.* Dubuque: Iowa: Brown and Benchmark, 1993.

Schinke, S.; B. Blythe; and L. Gilchrest. "Cognitive-Behavioral Prevention of Adolescent Pregnancy," *Journal of Counseling Psychology,* Vol. 28 (1981), 451–54.

School-Based Conflict Resolution Programs: A California Resource Guide. Sacramento: Sacramento County Office of Education, 1997.

School Health: Helping Children Learn. Alexandria, Va.: National School Boards Association, 1991.

Schools and Health: Our Nation's Investment. Edited by Diane Allensworth and others. Washington, D.C.: National Academy Press, 1997.

Second to None: A Vision of the New California High School. Sacramento: California Department of Education, 1992.

Seffrin, J. R. "The Comprehensive School Health Curriculum: Closing the Gap Between State-of-the-Art and State-of-the-Practice," *Journal of School Health,* Vol. 60, No. 4 (1990), 151–56.

Sipe, C., and others. *School-Based Programs for Adolescent Parents and Their Young Children: Overcoming Barriers and Challenges to Implementing Comprehensive School-Based Services in California and Across the Country.* Bala Cynwyd, Pa.: Center for Assessment and Policy Development, 1995.

Smith, Mark K. *Paulo Freire.* The Home of Informal Education Web site *<http://www.infed.org/thinkers/et-freir>*. 1997.

Springer, J. Fred. "Beyond the Magic Bullet: How We Can Achieve Science-Based Prevention," in *Getting Results, Update 1: Positive Youth Development: Research, Commentary, and Action.* Sacramento: California Department of Education, 1999.

The Surgeon General's Call to Action to Prevent Suicide. Washington, D.C.: United States Public Health Service, 1999.

Ten Leading Causes of Death, United States. Centers for Disease Control and Prevention Web site *<http://webapp.cdc.gov/sasweb/ncipc/leadcaus10.html>*. 2000.

Tobler, N. S. "Drug Prevention Programs Can Work: Research Findings," *Journal of Addictive Diseases,* Vol. 11, No. 3 (1992), 1–28.

Tobler, N. S., and H. H. Stratton. "Effectiveness of School-Based Drug Prevention Programs: A Meta-Analysis of the Research," *Journal of Primary Prevention,* Vol. 18, No. 1 (1997), 71–128.

Vaiana, Mary, and Ian Coulter. *The Oral Health of California's Children: Halting the Neglected Epidemic—California Children's Dental Health Initiative.* Oakland, Calif.: The Dental Health Foundation, 2000.

Vital Statistics of California, 1998. Sacramento: California Department of Health Services, 1999.

Vossekuil, B., and others. *Safe School Initiative: An Interim Report on the Prevention of Targeted Violence in Schools.* Washington, D.C.: U.S. Secret Service, National Threat Assessment Center, 2000.

Youth Risk Behavior Survey. Atlanta: Centers for Disease Control and Prevention, 1999.

Additional References and Resources

New resources in the field of school health have become available since the 1994 *Health Framework* was published. These resources provide a wealth of information, offering guidance on curriculum development and assessment and planning tools for developing the components of a coordinated school health system. The references and resources that follow are organized by category.

California Healthy Kids Resource Center

The California Healthy Kids Resource Center (HKRC) is a well-established resource for school health programs and related issues, providing up-to-date information on assessment, research, programs, training, and laws related to school health. Teachers, health professionals, and others who work with students may borrow HKRC materials at no charge.

California Healthy Kids Resource Center
313 W. Winton Avenue, Room 180
Hayward, CA 94544
(510) 670-4581; FAX (510) 670-4582
<http://www.hkresources.org>

Other Agencies

The following agencies offer guidance and resources relevant to school health programs:

Healthy Start and After-School Partnerships Program Office
California Department of Education
1430 N Street, Suite 6408
Sacramento, CA 95814
(916) 319-0923; FAX (916) 319-0221

National Association of State Boards of Education
277 South Washington Street, Suite 100
Alexandria, VA 22314
(704) 684-4000

National Institutes of Health
6601 Executive Boulevard, Room 8184
Bethesda, MD 20892
(301) 496-4000

Safe and Healthy Kids Program Office
California Department of Education
1430 N Street, Suite 6408
Sacramento, CA 95814
(916) 319-0920; FAX (916) 319-0218

School Health Connections Office
California Department of Education
1430 N Street, Suite 6408
Sacramento, CA 95814
(916) 319-0914; FAX (916) 445-7367

Youth Education and Partnerships Office
California Department of Education
1430 N Street, Suite 6408
Sacramento, CA 95814
(916) 319-0917; FAX (916) 319-0219

Planning Tools

The Centers for Disease Control and Prevention (CDC), the National Association of State Boards of Education, and the Council of Chief State School Officers offer planning tools for developing coordinated school health systems. The following documents are examples of those resources:

Bogden, J. F., and C. A. Vega-Matos. *Fit, Healthy, and Ready to Learn: A School Health Policy Guide.* Alexandria, Va.: National Association of State Boards of Education, 2000.

Guidelines for School and Community Programs to Promote Lifelong Physical Activity Among Young People. Atlanta: Centers for Disease Control and Prevention, 1997.

Guidelines for School Health Programs to Prevent Tobacco Use and Addiction. Atlanta: Centers for Disease Control and Prevention, 1994.

Guidelines for School Health Programs to Promote Lifelong Healthy Eating. Atlanta: Centers for Disease Control and Prevention, 1996.

School Health Index for Physical Activity, Healthy Eating, and a Tobacco-Free Lifestyle: A Self-Assessment and Planning Guide—Elementary School. Atlanta: Centers for Disease Control and Prevention, 2002. Copies of this document are available at no charge from CDC, telephone (888) 231-6405. The document can be downloaded from the CDC Web site at *<http://www.cdc.gov/nccdphp/dash/SHI/ elementary.htm>*.

School Health Index for Physical Activity, Healthy Eating, and a Tobacco-Free Lifestyle: A Self-Assessment and Planning Guide—Middle School/High School. Atlanta: Centers for Disease Control and Prevention, 2002. Copies of this document are available at no charge from CDC, telephone (888) 231-6405. The document can be downloaded from the CDC Web site at *<http://www.cdc.gov/nccdphp/dash/SHI/ middle_high.htm>*.

Publications

The following publications offer detailed information on coordinated school health programs:

Getting Results, Part 1: California Action Guide to Creating Safe and Drug-Free Schools and Communities. Sacramento: California Department of Education, 1998.

Getting Results, Part II: California Action Guide to Tobacco-Use Prevention Education. Sacramento: California Department of Education, 2000.

Getting Results, Update 1: Positive Youth Development: Research, Commentary, and Action. Sacramento: California Department of Education, 1999.

Getting Results, Update 2: Assessing the Effectiveness of Classroom-Based Prevention Programs. Sacramento: California Department of Education, 2001.

Getting Results, Update 3: Alcohol, Tobacco, Other Drug Use, and Violence Prevention: Research Update. Sacramento: California Department of Education, 2002.

Health Is Academic: A Guide to Coordinated School Health Programs. Edited by Eva Marx, Susan Frelick Wooley, and Daphne Northrop. New York: Teachers College Press, 1998.

This collection of essays by nationally known experts in their respective fields helps to define the theoretical and practical aspects of coordinated school health programs through a detailed examination of each of the eight components.

Schools and Health: Our Nation's Investment. Edited by Diane Allensworth and others. Washington, D.C.: National Academy Press, 1997.

This landmark report presents the findings and recommendations of the National Academy of Science, Institute of Medicine, regarding coordinated school health programs and systems.

Web Sites

Because many Web sites soon become outdated, only a few selected sites are listed in this section. Each of the following Web sites is updated regularly and contains links to other relevant Web sites:

California Center for Health Improvement's Health Policy Coach
 <http://www.healthpolicycoach.org>

California Department of Education, School Health Connections Office
 <http://www.cde.ca.gov/cyfsbranch/lsp/health>

California Department of Education, Safe and Healthy Kids Program Office
 <http://www.cde.ca.gov/healthykids>

California Department of Health Services
 <http://www.dhs.cahwnet.gov>

California Department of Health Services, School Health Connections Office
 <http://www.mch.dhs.ca.gov/programs/shc/shc.htm>

California Department of Mental Health
  <http://www.dmh.cahwnet.gov>

California Healthy Kids Resource Center
  <http://www.hkresources.org>

California Healthy Kids Survey
  <http://www.wested.org/hks>

California School Boards Association
  <http://www.csba.org>

California Student Survey
  <http://www.safestate.org/index.cfm?navID=254>

California Tobacco Survey Results
  <http://www.dhs.ca.gov/tobacco/documents/CTS99FinalReport.pdf>

California Youth Tobacco Survey Instrument
  <http://www.dhs.ca.gov/tobacco/documents/LPEdhscyts99.pdf>

Centers for Disease Control and Prevention, Division of Adolescent
  and School Health
  <http://www.cdc.gov/nccdphp/dash>

Education Training Research Associates
  <http://www.etr.org>

Monitoring the Future
  <http://www.monitoringthefuture.org>

National Association of State Boards of Education
  <http://www.nasbe.org>

National Institutes of Health
  <http://www.nih.gov>

National Strategy for Suicide Prevention
  <http://www.mentalhealth.org/suicideprevention>

Official California Legislative Information
  <http://www.leginfo.ca.gov>

School Health Policies and Programs Study
  <http://www.cdc.gov/nccdphp/dash/shpps/index.htm>

Search Institute
  <http://www.search-institute.org>

Tufts University, Nutrition Navigator
  <http://www.navigator.tufts.edu>

U.S. Department of Health and Human Services, Healthy
  People 2010 Initiative
  <http://www.healthypeople.gov>

Women, Infants, and Children Supplemental Nutrition Program
  <http://www.wicworks.ca.gov>

Youth Risk Behavior Surveillance System
  <http://www.cdc.gov/nccdphp/dash/yrbs>

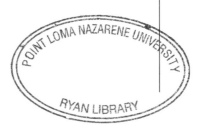

01-024 103-0045-01 6-03 25M

UNION LABEL OSP 03 69471